Deskercise!

The Workplace Workout

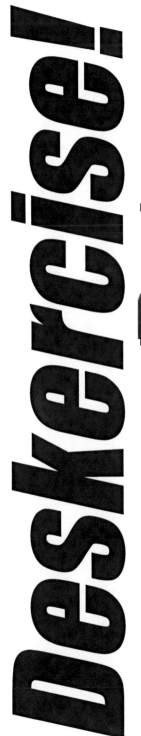

THE WORKPLACE WORKOUT

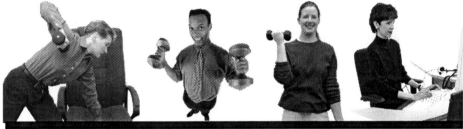

A Revolutionary Exercise Program You Can Do Right At Your Desk!

DR. TODD M BERNTSON

FOREWORD BY DR. JACQUELINE BURNS

Disclaimer

The information in this book is intended for educational use only and should not be construed as medical advice. You should consult with your physician before starting any exercise regimen, including this one. If you feel shortness of breath, heaviness in your chest or dizziness, stop exercising immediately and seek care.

Center Path Media, Inc.
14859 Embry Path
Apple Valley, MN 55124

Library of Congress Control Number: 2004094997

ISBN 0-9724022-1-7

Printed in the United States of America

∞ The paper used in this publication meets the minimum requirements of the American National Standard for Information Services - Permanence of Paper for Printed Library Materials, ANSI Z39.48-1984.

Order information:

To order additional copies of this title, please use the form located on the back page of this book. A quantity discount of this title is also available. Inquiries should be addressed to Center Path Media Inc. at the above address or via email: orders@centerpathmedia.com.

This book is dedicated to my wife Monique.

Foreword

Everyone knows that exercise is important for good health. Study after study has shown that exercise is effective at decreasing pain, reducing stress, improving immune function, lowering blood pressure, improving cardiac function, boosting energy, improving sleep and maintaining a healthy bodyweight. The fact remains that although most people are aware of how important exercise is to their health, they still do not exercise the way that they should.

Many people are under the mistaken impression that in order for an exercise program to be effective, it has to be difficult, time consuming and require a lot of equipment. And because of our increasingly busy schedules, most of us do not make the time to exercise and develop a healthier lifestyle. What most people need is a quick and simple way to get the exercise necessary to maintain good health. That is where Deskercise fits in.

Deskercise is an effective exercise and stretching program that doesn't require a lot of time and the only equipment you need is a desk, a chair, a pair of dumbbells and a little motivation. I have used this exercise program and other information in this book successfully within my own practice. The strength of this program is that it takes only minutes per day, can be done virtually anywhere, and will improve the quality of your life.

Even after working for years as a chiropractor, I am still amazed at how powerful exercise can be as a healing tool. In addition to the obvious benefit of increasing strength, it is also critical to the maintenance of optimal posture, mobility, strength and coordination. Optimal posture prevents chronic muscle strain, improved mobility results in less pain and better balance, muscle strength reduces muscle tension, and good coordination allows you to be as active as you want without injuring yourself. After only a short time of doing the Deskercise program, you should begin to notice an improvement in how you feel.

If you are looking for a simple way to improve your health and feel better, then this is the book for you. Dr. Berntson has a unique ability to easily explain how the human body is designed and how the average occupational duties cause us to work against this design. He has taken the most important stretches and exercises for good health and incorporated them into an easy to use system that you can perform at your desk. It is not necessary for you to spend an hour a day at the gym and you do not need expensive, specialized equipment. Dr. Berntson has developed a program that utilizes gravity and your own body weight to improve muscle tone and function. This makes your muscles and joints smarter, stronger and able to withstand daily stresses.

The Deskercise program that Dr. Berntson has developed takes only minutes per day, requires little or no equipment and the pictures and explanations are easily understood. While I recommend that you consult with a Doctor of Chiropractic to find out whether such a program is right for you, I hope that you will seriously consider taking this small step toward improving your life.

- Dr. Jacqueline S. Burns
Eagan, Minnesota

Preface

Ergonomics, the study of the relationship between workers and their work environment, began to gain popularity in the late 1980s as businesses recognized how much the physical work environment impacted the health and productivity of its workers. Until recently, most of the focus has been on minimizing occupational stress through improved workspace design; including improved chair design, customizable and angled keyboards, better lighting, adjustable work surfaces and safety training. These advances have resulted in an overall improvement in employee performance and a decrease in job-related injuries.

However, ergonomics has not proven to be the magic bullet that most people expected. High health care expenses, absenteeism, occupational injuries and an overall loss of performance are still epidemic in the workplace, despite correct workspace design. This is not due to the failure of ergonomics, *per se*, but rather to the fact that ergonomics covers only one side of the health equation. The other side, which has been largely overlooked until very recently, is the active physical component - exercise.

A few companies have implemented exercise-based workplace wellness

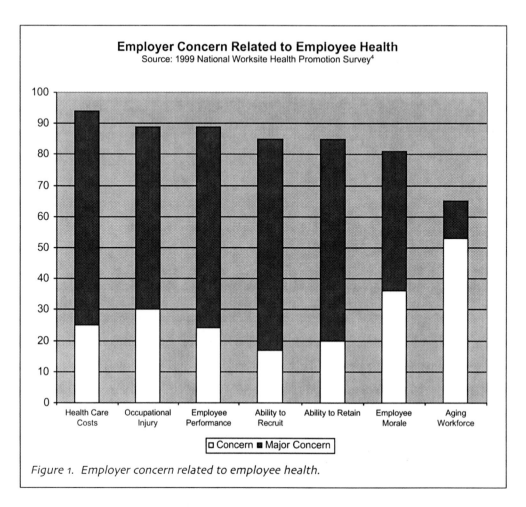

Figure 1. Employer concern related to employee health.

programs to actively counteract the detrimental physical effects of job stress, and the results from follow-up studies have been remarkable. Companies such as Coors, Steel-Case, the Municipal Employees of Toronto, Canada Life Assurance, DuPont and Control Data have enjoyed a dramatic improvement in productivity and morale and an equally impressive decrease in employee turnover, health care costs, work-related injury and absenteeism - the very issues that most companies identified as major employee health concerns (Figure 1). As a matter of fact, it is estimated that the average organization realizes a $3.00 to $5.00 return on every dollar they spend on exercise-based wellness programs.[1-8]

For example, data from a cost-benefit study on a fitness program sponsored by BC Hydro showed a $1.2 million reduction in annual sick leave costs, $97,000 reduction in annual accident costs, $35,000 reduction in their Workers' Compensation insurance premiums, productivity gains of $919,000 and a 60% reduction in employee turnover.[2]

Steelcase, a large furniture maker, rated as one of the top 100 places to work by Fortune Magazine, enjoyed a significant drop in the number of job-related injuries - up to 50% in one department - after just three months of implementing a 20 minute stretching program to help employees warm up before starting work.[7]

The Staywell program implemented by Control Data Corporation in Minneapolis, Minnesota, has saved the company an estimated $1.8 million dollars over a six-year period as the result of reduced absenteeism.[7]

In addition to the physical benefits, exercise has been shown to improve psychological functioning, decrease emotional stress and to elevate mood. Studies reveal that physically active persons are more likely to be better emotionally adjusted,[9] perform better on tests of cognitive functioning,[10] exhibit reduced cardiovascular responses to stress,[11] and report fewer symptoms of anxiety and depression.[12] Exercise also improves self-confidence and self-esteem[13] and decreases the cardiovascular responses to mental stress.[14-15]

Worksite health programs, which include exercise, benefit companies by decreasing health care costs, decreasing occupational injuries, improving employee performance, boosting morale and decreasing employee turnover and absenteeism. It also helps companies improve their image and good-will between employees and management, thereby helping them to attract and retain the finest workers.

Although most of the evidence supporting the exercise-based worksite wellness programs comes from larger corporations, there is ample evidence that small companies can enjoy comparable benefits as well. Although specific outcomes depend somewhat on the nature of the business, the most extensively documented and widely experienced benefits are the reduction of employee health risks and reduced absenteeism. The savings from these reductions are usually significant. Most companies have found that the savings from reduced absenteeism alone more than offsets the cost of a health promotion program.[7]

The Deskercise program outlined in this book was designed to be a non-invasive way for employees to enjoy the benefits of better health through exercise, while keeping time and equipment requirements to a minimum. It is written specifically for the individual employee who may not work for a company offering a comprehensive worksite health program. But it is just as useful to a medium or large sized corporation as an integral part of a larger workplace health promotion program.

References

1.   Shephard, Roy J. Twelve Years Experience of a Fitness Program for the Salaried Employees of a Toronto Life Assurance Company. *American Journal of Health Promotion* 6(4) 292-301 March/April 1992

2.   Shephard, Roy J. Do Work-Site Exercise and Health Programs Work? The Physician and Sportsmedicine Online - February 1999

3. Ten Research Studies You Can't Afford to Ignore, Part IV. Worksite Health 1998; 5(3): 23-27.

4. 1999 National Worksite Health Promotion Survey: Conducted by the Association for Worksite Health Promotion; William M. Mercer, Incorporated; and the U.S. Department of Health and Human Services, Office of Disease Prevention and Health Promotion; 1999.

5. Chapman LS. Proof Positive: An Analysis of the Cost-Effectiveness of Worksite Wellness. 4th ed. Seattle, WA: Summex Corporation; 1999.

6. Chapman LS. Clearing Up the Productivity "Fog". The Art of Health Promotion1999; 3(5): 1-12.

7. Aldana SG. Financial Impact of Worksite Health Promotion and Methodological Quality of the Evidence. The Art of Health Promotion1998; 2(1).

8. Gemignani J. Best practices that boost productivity. Bus Health1998; 16(3): 37-42.

9.   Eysenck HJ, Nias DKB, Cox DN. Sport and personality. *Adv Behav Res Ther.* 1982;4:1-56.

10.   Spirduso WW. Physical fitness, aging, and psychomotor speed: a review. *J Gerontol.* 1980;35:850-865.

11.   Crews DJ, Landers DM. A meta-analytic review of aerobic fitness and reactivity to psychosocial stressors. *Med Sci Sports Exerc.* 1987;19:S114-S120.

12.   Lobstein DD, Mosbacher BJ, Ismail AH. Depression as a powerful discriminator between physically active and sedentary middle-aged men. *J Psychosom Res.* 1983;27:69-76.

13.   Folkins CH, Sime WE. Physical fitness training and mental health. *Am J Psychol.* 1981;36:373-389.

14.   Blumenthal JA, Fredrikson M, Kuhn CM, Ulmer RL, Walsh-Riddle M, Appelbaum M. Aerobic exercise reduces levels of cardiovascular and sympathoadrenal responses to mental stress in subjects without prior evidence of myocardial ischemia. *Am J Cardiol.* 1990;65:93-98.

15. Blumenthal JA, Emery CF, Walsh MA, Cox DR, Kuhn CM, Williams RB, Williams RS. Exercise training in healthy type A middle-aged men: effects on behavioral and cardiovascular responses. *Psychosom Med.* 1988;50:418-433.

Acknowledgements

I would like first and foremost to thank you for buying this book. All of the blood, sweat and tears that went into creating this book would have been for naught without good people like you to read it. I would like to thank Dr. Joseph Sweere from Northwestern Health Sciences University, Dr. Angela Gear, Elizabeth Auppl from the International Association of Chiropractic Occupational Health Consultants, Judy Robinson and Monique Berntson for their editorial help in the preparation of this manuscript. Their help was invaluable. I would like to thank Dr. Jacqueline Burns from South Lexington Chiropractic for taking the time to write the foreword. I need to offer a big thanks to all of those who were willing to take their time to demonstrate the exercises and stretches in front of the camera: Monique Berntson, Dr. Jacqueline Burns, Scott Conrad, Peter Guenther, Jason Kuebelbeck, Nancy McNulty and Laura Vander Heyden. Last, but not least, I would like to thank the gang at Barnes & Noble for allowing me to take over a corner of their café while I wrote this book.

Thanks Everyone!!!

Table of Contents

I Introduction: The Wellness Win-Win

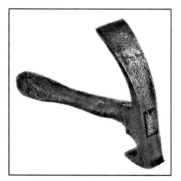

When I was a kid, I learned two things about tools from watching my father. The first was that most tools, regardless of their shape, could be used for just about any purpose: screwdrivers could be used to pound in nails, pliers could be used to drive in a screw, a screwdriver could be used to drill a hole in the wall, and a metal t-square could be used to chop ice. The second thing I learned was that my dad's tools didn't last very long. Whenever a tool broke, my father would exclaim "what a piece of junk," as if it was the tool's fault that it broke.

It wasn't until years later that I figured out the reason my dad's tools always broke. He wasn't using them in the way they were designed to be used. When he struck the head of a nail over and over again with the plastic handle of a screwdriver, he created a stress on the tool that it could not bear for long. Consequently, the handle would eventually break and he would speak a few choice words about the cheap quality of the tool. But it wasn't that his tools were 'cheap' or 'junk.' It was the way he was using them that caused them to break.

The fact is that most of us do the same thing to our body when we go to work every day. When we sit and work at a desk all day, we use our body in a way that it was not designed to be used. It is important to understand that the human body is simply a complex tool which was never designed to withstand the stresses of sitting at a desk for several hours every day. Consequently, if we don't take the time to counteract these stresses, our body will eventually break down and we will experience dysfunction and pain.

The vast majority of headaches, pain in the lower back, upper back, legs, arms, wrists and hands are merely the inevitable consequences of stressing the body in ways it was not designed to be stressed. To help you understand why having a 'cushy' job is so hard on the body, let's go back in time and look at how the human body was designed.

The Design of the Human Body

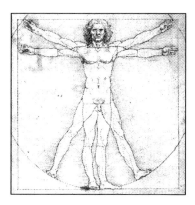

Estimates are that the 'modern' human body as we know it first appeared about 150,000 years ago. To put this into perspective, imagine that the time humans have lived on this planet is equivalent to one hour on a clock. Each passing second would be roughly equivalent to 187 years. If this were the case, the fall of the Roman Empire would have occurred only eleven seconds ago, Galileo Galilei would have discovered that the Earth revolved around the sun only five seconds ago, and the industrial revolution, harking the first appearance of desk jobs for average people, only occurred about one second ago. During the previous 3,599 seconds of the hour – or 149,813 years – people lived very physically demanding lives, performing daily manual labor by gathering nuts and roots, hunting, chopping wood, carrying water, walking all day and building everything by hand.

In the final one second, people are suddenly riding in cars, sitting all day at desks, watching television, surfing the internet, playing video games and eating way too much food. Living with such a restricted activity level is the human equivalent of using the handle of a screwdriver to pound in a nail. Our bodies were simply not designed for this kind of lifestyle.

Unfortunately, most of us just can't quit our desk jobs and go back to being primitive hunters. But we can integrate specific activities into our daily routine which will counteract the stresses of working at a desk job. That is exactly what the Deskercise program is designed to do.

Introducing the Deskercise Program

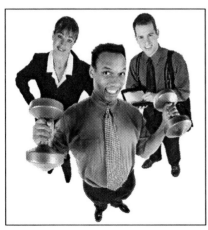

The Deskercise program is an exercise and stretching routine designed to help rebuild the body's healthy posture, mobility, strength and coordination. Although this book was written primarily for those who work at desk jobs, the information in this book is valid for anyone who wants to improve their health and how they feel.

The exercises and stretches included in this program are specially selected and designed so they can be performed within the confines of an average work-space in only a few minutes per day and require very little extra equipment. All you need is a desk, a chair, a pair of dumbbells and a good attitude to get a full body workout and counteract the deliterious effects of workplace stress.

As in most endeavors, what you get out of the Deskercise program will depend on what you put into it. The more you push yourself to do the exercises and stretches every day and to lift enough weight to challenge your muscles, the greater the results. If you only look at your exercise chart twice – once when you first hang it on the wall in your office and again when you take it down after you discover it still hanging there six months later – you will not experience much of an improvement. But if you do the exercises and stretches on a regular basis, you will experience a dramatic improvement in how you feel. Most people experience increased energy, improved muscle strength and decreased physical pain and are able to think more clearly, sleep better and have an improved overall sense of well-being.

With skyrocketing health care costs, the Deskercise program is a wellness win-win for everyone. For you, a simple workout like the Deskercise program will improve your physical strength, stamina and general health. It will help improve your focus at work, help increase your job satisfaction and improve your overall quality of life.

For your employer, the Deskercise program can help boost productivity, reduce the costs associated with absenteeism and help to reduce turnover. It can also improve on-the-job decision-making and time utilization and improve employee morale. So if you are ready to improve your health, quality of life and your effectiveness at work, let's get Deskercising!

Strategies for Success

The sad truth is that most people find it difficult to stay on an exercise program for a meaningful length of time. The reason is that people are creatures of habit. Changing those habits is sometimes hard, but it is not impossible. Those who are successful at changing their unhealthy habits to healthier ones tend to do four things: they don't get discouraged when they don't see results at first, they schedule their workout time into their daily schedule, they start small and gradually build up their level of exercise and they keep track of their progress.

Do Not Get Discouraged

Changing your lifestyle habits is like being a child who is learning to walk. Just as when you were a young child who had never walked before, you are attempting to switch to a lifestyle that is unfamiliar to you. It is normal for new habits to require a tremendous amount of mental effort at first. But over time, just as walking became natural to you as a child, your new healthier lifestyle will begin to feel natural to you. It is important to give yourself a break if you don't do everything perfect at first. Try to see yourself again as a baby learning to walk and don't worry if you stumble and don't do your exercises for a few days or weeks. Just start again and eventually, your habits will change.

Schedule Your Workout Time

If you are like most people, you probably have a busy schedule. But, just as you set aside time every day to work, to shower and dress every morning and time each day to spend with your family, you need to set aside a small amount of time each day to take care of your physical health.

Some people use the excuse that they just don't have the time to exercise. This is simply not true. Everyone has the exact same amount of time each day - 24 hours. Each day we make decisions on how we will spend that 24 hours based on what we value. What these people are really saying when they claim to not have enough time for exercise is that they don't value exercising as much as they value doing something else, such as watching television, shopping, or surfing the net. There are people who go to school, work full-time, raise children and still have enough time in their schedule to exercise regularly. It's all just a matter of making your health a priority.

Start Small, Build Gradually

When starting any exercise program, it is important to start small and build up the intensity over time. It takes time for the body to ramp up its metabolism and strength. If you try to do too much too quickly, you may end up straining your muscles. It's better to work out at a reduced intensity for the first two to three weeks before working out at full intensity. As your body changes and becomes stronger, you will be able to increase the intensity of your workout with a much lower risk of injury.

It is important to remember when beginning an exercise program that the only person you are competing against is yourself. You should never feel embarrassed or bad in any way because of how much or little you can do. If you are like many people who are beginning an exercise program, you may be afraid of looking like you don't know what you are doing, especially around people who work out regularly and are in great shape. In actuality, those who are in great shape will understand exactly what you are trying to do for yourself and will admire you for your committment to get in shape. You will find that those who are in the best shape will be your greatest cheerleaders and will usually help you in any way they can. If you know or work with people who have the kind of physique you admire, you should get to know them, tell them that you are beginning an exercise program and use them as a resource when you have questions or concerns.

Measure Your Progress

Measuring and keeping track of your progress is important for a number of reasons. First, keeping track of your progress helps build momentum. Being able to see how your efforts are paying off creates excitement and enthusiasm for continuing with your exercises and stretches. This excitement helps to motivate you during times when you just don't feel like exercising.

Second, keeping track of your progress allows you to see what works for you. Are your muscles getting stronger? Are you more flexible than you were? Do you have better posture? Is your body weight improving? Unless you have a way to measure these, you can't be sure. But if you keep a regular record of your progress, it is easy to see where you are making gains and where you are not. This gives you valuable information about where to make changes in order to improve your exercise and stretching routine.

Third, keeping track of your progress helps keep you honest. When it comes to our bodies, all of us have a tendency to misjudge ourselves; sometimes by a lot. People like to see themselves in a positive way, so we tend to underestimate potentially negative aspects of our body. Measuring ourselves objectively and keeping a written record of our progress keeps us honest with ourselves.

1 Your Bones, Joints, Muscles and Nerves

Bones & Joints:
The Framework of the Body

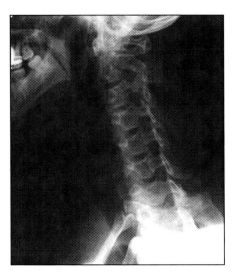

The human skeleton is made up of more than 200 bones which are connected by joints. Your bones are responsible for creating your body's general shape, they serve to protect your internal organs and to manufacture blood cells. Each of your bones is made up of two compounds: a protein meshwork of collagen and a salt of calcium called hydroxyapatite.

The collagen fibers which make up the basic structure of your bones gives them a great deal of resilience and resistance to breaking when twisted, bent or impacted. It is actually the loss of this collagen meshwork and not just a loss of calcium that is responsible for the bone weakness associated with conditions such as osteoporosis. The other component of bone, hydroxyapatite, is a crystalline calcium salt which is integrated into the collagen meshwork. Hydroxyapatite is responsible for giving the bones rigidity and resistance to crushing under pressure.

Bones can be compared to steel-reinforced concrete, where the collagen meshwork acts much like the steel meshwork in the concrete and the hydroxyapatite acts much like the concrete which surrounds the steel. Together they form a very tough, resilient and rigid framework upon which the rest of the body is supported. But, because your bones are rigid and do not bend, you would not be able to move if it were not for your joints.

Joints are much more than simply a place where the ends of two bones meet. They are very complicated systems of ligaments, tendons, membranes and cartilage that allow the bones to move in a smooth, stable and controlled way. Joints are designed in a wide variety of ways depending on their function and the particular stresses they have to endure. For example, the joints between your sternum (breastbone) and your ribs are simple joints consisting only of fibrous collagen. They are designed to be simple because the front part of your rib cage does not have to move very much in relation to your sternum. The shoulder joint on the other hand is an extremely complex joint that requires a whole host of muscles, ligaments and tendons all working in concert with each other in order to move properly. If any one of the muscles or other structures of the shoulder are damaged, pain, instability or loss of function may result.

Later in this chapter we will discuss a particular set of joints that are especially important to people who work at desk jobs; those are the joints of the spine. But first let's take a look at your muscles.

Muscles:
The Engines of Movement

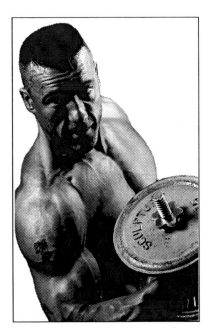

There are more than 650 muscles in your body which have only one purpose – to create movement. While your bones are what give your body its framework, it is the muscles that give your body motion. There are more than three times the number of muscles in your body as there are bones, and each one of these muscles fills a particular role in creating movement. Like bones, your muscles also contain a lot of collagen for strength and resilience. But instead of calcium salts, muscles contain a specialized type of cell which has the unique ability to contract when stimulated by the nervous system.

There are actually three types of muscle in the body - smooth muscle, cardiac muscle and striated muscle (also called skeletal muscle). Smooth muscle is found surrounding the organs of the digestive tract as well as the arteries. In the digestive tract, smooth muscle is responsible for moving the food we eat through our digestive system, while the smooth muscle which surrounds the arteries helps the regulation of blood flow throughout the body. Unlike skeletal muscles, smooth muscles are involuntary muscles, meaning that we do not have conscious control over them.

Cardiac muscle, as its name implies, is found only in the heart. What differentiates cardiac muscle from all other muscle in the body is the fact that it rhythmically contracts on its own, regardless of stimulation by the nervous system. As a matter of fact, if two independent cardiac cells, each rhythmically contracting to their own beat are put in contact with each other, they will begin beating in unison. And it's a good thing, otherwise our heart wouldn't beat very regularly.

The third type of muscle is skeletal muscle. This is the type of muscle that we can consciously control and the type of muscle that is of most interest to us in the Deskercise program because it is the type of muscle responsible for our posture and movement. Every skeletal muscle attaches to at least two different bones and as they contract, they draw the bones together, using the joints as hinges, allowing controlled movement to take place.

Take for example the elbow joint. Compared to some of the other joints in the body, such as the shoulder or hip, the elbow is a relatively simple hinge joint. Yet, there are more than a dozen muscles which cross the elbow joint - all of which contribute to the elbow's normal movement. If any of these muscles do not fire in a highly coordinated fashion, or if some of the muscles are tighter than they should be, or if some of the muscles are weaker than they should be, abnormal joint function and pain will likely result.

Abnormal posture and joint motion resulting from weak, spasmed or incoordinated muscles is so common in people who do their work seated at a desk that it is rare for them not to be present. That is, unless they do the necessary exercises to counteract the effects of working at a desk job. Before we discuss what these exercises are and how to do them correctly, let's continue our discussion of body mechanics by looking at the nervous system.

The Nervous System:
The Master Controller

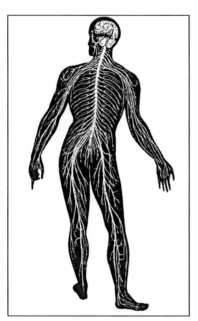

The nervous system is made up of trillions of highly-specialized individual nerve cells, each of which communicate with hundreds or thousands of other nerve cells through tiny electrical pulses, and is comprised of two major systems. One is called the central nervous system which includes your brain and spinal cord, and the other is called the peripheral nervous system which includes the nerves that run from your spine to all areas of the body. The nervous system is called the master controller as it is responsible for the control of all major body functions including our senses, movement and balance, as well as the regulations of all body functions.

There are three types of nerves that are important to our discussion. These are called pain nerves, motor nerves and postural nerves, or more correctly, proprioceptors. Pain nerves do just what their name implies - they allow us to feel pain. Whenever something in our body hurts, it is because the pain nerves in the area are being stimulated and sending signals to the brain to create the sensation of pain.

Motor nerves are responsible for controlling our movement by stimulating muscles to contract. The fact that you are able to hold this book in your hands right now is because these motor nerves are contracting the muscles in your hands and arms. If these nerves aren't able to function correctly, it can result in weakness, or even paralysis, in the muscles they control.

The third type of nerve is the proprioceptor, or what we will simply call the postural nerves. These nerves are responsible for sending information to the brain about where your body is and what it's doing. For example, if you close your eyes and hold your arm out to your side, you can tell exactly where your arm is even though you can't see it because the postural nerves of the arm and upper back tell the brain where your arm is. Many people have discovered what happens when their postural nerves aren't working correctly after they have had too much to drink. Alcohol partially disrupts your postural nerves, making it difficult to touch your finger to your nose when your eyes are closed, or walk a straight line with your eyes open.

In the next section, we will be pulling all of this information on bones, joints, muscles and nerves together in a discussion about body mechanics.

The Four Pillars
Of Body Mechanics

As we have discussed in the previous sections of this chapter, the human body is an amazingly complex system of bones, joints, muscles, and nerves, designed to work together to accomplish one thing: movement. Movement is one of the defining characteristics that separates us from plants, bacteria and fungus. Everything about the human body is designed with movement in mind – nerve fibers stimulate the muscles to contract, muscles contract to move the bones, bones move around joints, and the nervous system controls it all.

As a matter of fact, research has shown that movement is so critical to our body's health that a lack of movement has a detrimental affect on everything from digestion, to our emotional state, immune function, our ability to concentrate, how well we sleep and even to how long we live. The bottom line is that if your lifestyle does not include enough movement, your body cannot function efficiently. Consequently, three things will happen: first, you will not be as physically healthy and will suffer from a wide variety of physical ailments, ranging from headaches to high blood pressure. Second, you will not be as productive in your life because of reduced energy levels and the ability to mentally focus. Third, because you have less energy, your activity level will tend to drop off even further over time, creating a downward spiral of reduced energy and less activity until you get to a point where even the demands of a sedentary job leave you physically exhausted by the end of the day.

The Deskercise program was created to help combat the effects just described - a condition referred to as deconditioning - and to do so within the tight time constraints under which most of us live. But before we get into the specifics of the exercises, let's take a look at the four important aspects of body mechanics: posture, motion, strength and coordination. These are the Four Pillars of Body Mechanics.

Pillar One: Posture

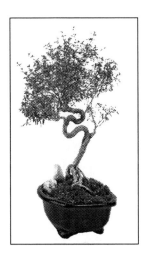

The ancient Japanese art form of growing Bonsai trees is fascinating. They are essentially normal shrubs that have been consistently stressed in a particular way for a long time to create a posture which would never be found in nature. Depending on how the tree is stressed while it grows, it may end up looking like a miniature version of a full-sized tree, or it may end up looking like a wild tangle of branches with twists and loops.

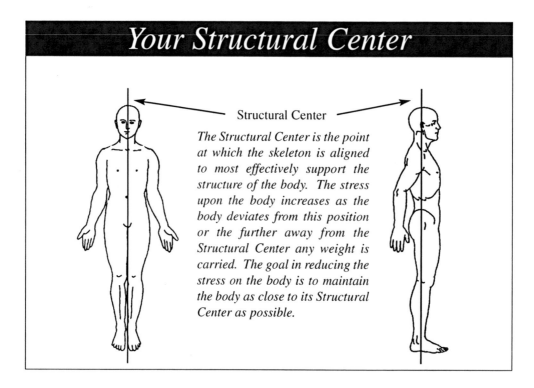

Your Structural Center

Structural Center

The Structural Center is the point at which the skeleton is aligned to most effectively support the structure of the body. The stress upon the body increases as the body deviates from this position or the further away from the Structural Center any weight is carried. The goal in reducing the stress on the body is to maintain the body as close to its Structural Center as possible.

Every day in my practice, I see the human equivalent of Bonsai trees walk through my door - people with an unnatural posture due to the continual daily stresses on their body. The most common unnatural posture is one that I call the Desk Distortion Posture where the individual's shoulders are rolled forward, they are hunched slightly and their head protrudes forward.

The most immediate problem with poor posture is that it creates a lot of chronic muscle tension as the weight of the head and upper body is having to be supported by the muscles instead of the bones. This effect becomes more pronounced the further your posture deviates from your Structural Center (See illustration).

To illustrate this idea further, think about carrying a briefcase. If you had to carry your briefcase with your arms outstretched in front of you, it would not take long before the muscles of your shoulders would be completely exhausted. This is because carrying the briefcase far away from your Structural

Center places an undue stress on your shoulder muscles. If you held the same briefcase down at your side, your muscles would not fatigue as quickly because the briefcase is closer to your Structural Center and the weight is, therefore, supported by the bones of the skeleton, rather than the muscles.

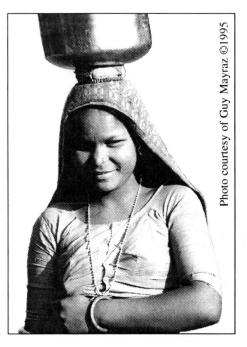

Photo courtesy of Guy Mayraz ©1995

In some parts of the world, women can carry big pots full of water from distant water sources back to their homes. They are able to carry these heavy pots a long distance without significant effort because they balance them on the top of their heads, thereby carrying them at their Structural Center and allowing the strength of their skeleton to bear the weight, rather than their muscles.

Correcting bad posture and the physical problems that result are accomplished by doing two things. The first is to eliminate as much 'bad' stress from your body as possible. Bad stress includes all the factors, habits or stressors that cause your body to deviate from your Structural Center. The most effective way to remove the bad stress on your job is by employing good ergonomics, such as adjusting your chair correctly and customizing your workspace to minimize the bad stress on your body. This is discussed in the next chapter.

The second is to apply 'good' stress on the body in an effort to move your posture back toward your Structural Center. Getting your body back to its Structural Center by improving your posture is critically important to improving how you feel. The only way to accomplish this is through specific exercises and stretches which are covered in detail in this book.

Pillar Two: Mobility

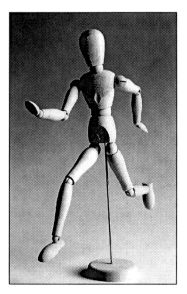

Imagine waking up one morning with a frozen shoulder where you couldn't move your upper arm more than a few inches in any direction. How much would that impact your ability to do your job? How much would that affect your ability to drive your car or even to dress yourself? How much would that affect your ability to concentrate on anything other than your shoulder? Obviously, if your shoulder did not move correctly, it would have a dramatic impact on your life. Well, the same is true with mobility in every part of your body. If things aren't moving the way they are supposed to move, it will have a negative impact on your ability to function at work, take care of the demands of everyday life and even your ability to concentrate.

Over the years, I have had a number of patients come into my clinic with severe low back pain who stated that their pain came on suddenly when they did something as simple as bend down to pet their cat, put on their socks, or pick up the newspaper. Just about everyone would agree that a person's body should be able to handle something as simple as bending over to pick up a newspaper or putting on their socks, right? So what happened?

In every one of these cases, we found that many of the joints in their body were barely moving at all; they were 'all locked up.' When the joints in one area of the body do not move the way they should, other areas of the body are forced to move more than they were designed to in an effort to compensate

Compensation for a Loss of Motion

Compensating Joint   Stuck Joint   Compensating Joint

When one joint is stuck, the joints around it have to move more than they are supposed to move, leading to inflammation, swelling and pain.

for the area that is not moving. This creates a significant stress on the areas that are having to pick up the slack of the joints that aren't moving so well. This soon leads to pain and inflammation. At the same time, the areas that don't have normal movement will slowly worsen as the muscles continue to tighten, the joints stick together and the ligaments and tendons shorten. This leaves the body in a very unstable condition and if left unchecked, this process will continue until the body can hardly move at all and the person suffers flare-ups of pain at the slightest provocation.

Most of us have seen people who have lost most of their normal mobility; they look like their whole body has been starched stiff whenever they try to move around. This is especially prevalent among the elderly. Contrary to popular belief, this is not the inevitable effect of aging, rather it is the inevitable effect of not maintaining the body's mobility through exercise, stretching and chiropractic care. There are a lot of people in their 60s, 70s or even older, who are stronger and more flexible than the average person in their 30s. One of those people is pictured in this book performing the Stiff-Leg Deadlifts.

Maintaining mobility is critical in order to live free from pain and disability. Maintaining good mobility is not difficult, but it does not happen on its own.

Just as in developing a good posture, it is necessary that you perform specific exercises and stretches to keep your muscles, ligaments and tendons flexible and healthy. In addition, it is necessary that all of the joints in your body are kept moving correctly as well. Although this can be achieved to a great degree through the exercises and stretches in this book, most people also find routine chiropractic care to be very beneficial.

Pillar Three: Strength

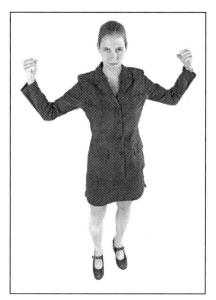

Strong muscles keep your body upright and allow you to move. Good muscle strength and balance are critical for proper posture and to minimize muscle tension. Your muscles function much like the wires that hold up a tall radio or television antenna. If the wires are equally strong on all sides, the antenna will stand up straight. If one of the wires becomes weak or breaks, the antenna will either lean to the side or collapse. The same is true with your body. If the muscles on all sides of your spine are balanced and strong, your body will stand up straight and strong. Unfortunately, most

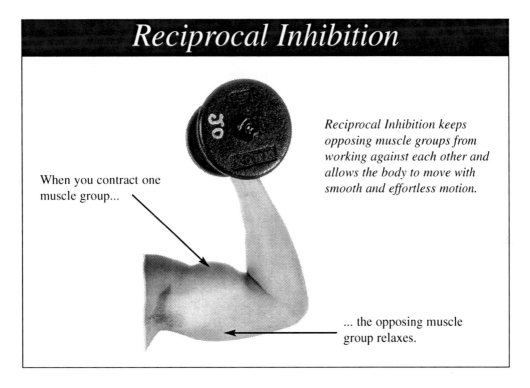

Reciprocal Inhibition

When you contract one muscle group...

Reciprocal Inhibition keeps opposing muscle groups from working against each other and allows the body to move with smooth and effortless motion.

... the opposing muscle group relaxes.

people don't have balanced and strong muscles. The reason for this gets back to exercise.

Muscles are very efficient at getting stronger or weaker in response to the demands placed on them. Since most of us sit at a desk, drive a car and sit on the sofa at home, many of our muscles are not challenged. Consequently, they become weak. At the same time, the muscles that are constantly used throughout the day become strong. This imbalance of muscle strength contributes to poor posture and chronic muscle tension. Left unchecked, muscle imbalances tend to get worse, not better, because of a phenomenon called *"Reciprocal Inhibition."*

Reciprocal Inhibition literally means *"shutting down the opposite."* Simply put, for all of the muscles that move your body in one direction, there are opposing muscles that move the body in the opposite direction. In order to keep these muscles from working against each other, when the body contracts one muscle group, it forces the opposing group to relax – it *shuts down the opposite* muscles. This becomes important to people who work at a desk, because all day long the same muscles on the front side of the body are used. This means that all day long the body is essentially shutting down the opposite muscles in the upper back. Over time, the muscles in the upper back become very weak because they are not being worked like the muscles in the front. As we will see in the next section, this becomes a real problem and contributes to poor posture and chronic muscle spasms and pain.

The easiest way to correct this imbalance is to do specific exercises which will increase the strength of the back muscles. Once the muscles in the back are strong and balanced with the muscles in the front side of your body, the tightness and poor posture disappear.

Pillar Four: Coordination

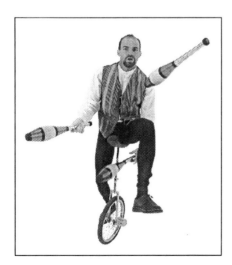

Jason was a powerlifter who was suffering from shoulder pain. I took x-rays, did all of the normal tests in an attempt to figure out what was wrong with his shoulders, but everything turned up normal. He was young, healthy, had incredible strength, great flexibility and no specific injury to the shoulders. Since the shoulder is a very mobile and unstable joint, I knew that if all of its muscles were not contracting in the correct order or with the right amount of tension, the result would be increased mechanical stress of the shoulder joint, ultimately resulting in pain.

I prescribed a series of very simple, lightweight exercises for him to do on a daily basis for the purpose of re-establishing normal shoulder coordination. The results were immediate and profound. Not only did his pain completely disappear, but his ability to bench press improved. It turned out that Jason's only problem was that his muscles were not coordinated correctly. Although posture, joint mobility and muscle strength are all important, they are not the whole story. We also must have coordinated control over our muscles and joints if we want to enjoy good body mechanics.

Healthy coordination is simply the result of using the body in the manner in which it was designed. Exercises such as walking, swimming, rock climbing, yoga, pilates, bicycling, martial arts and body building all help to improve muscle coordination, whereas working at a desk, reading and watching television do the opposite. Without realizing it, most people are in a dramatic state of muscle incoordination. This occurs simply because they sit for many hours every day and do not perform exercises on a regular basis that will work to keep all of the muscles in their body properly coordinated. This muscular incoordination contributes to muscle tightness, restricted movement and joint pain.

Got All That?

In this chapter we discussed the four components of the neuromusculoskeletal system; namely the bones and joints which serve as the framework for the body, the muscles which are responsible for movement and the nervous system which is responsible for controlling it all.

We also discussed the Four Pillars of Body Mechanics - posture, mobility, strength and coordination - and why each of these are important. You learned that when your posture deviates from your Structural Center, your muscles tighten up, resulting in pain and decreased mobility. You learned that once you begin to lose mobility, it usually continues to worsen unless you perform specific exercises and stretches to re-establish normal motion. You learned that muscles will either become stronger or weaker depending on how much they get used and that muscular imbalances will often lead to chronic muscle spasms and pain. Finally, you learned about the important role of coordination in acheiving good body mechanics.

The exercise and stretching program presented in this book is specifically designed to address each and every one of these issues to ensure that you develop a healthier posture, improved mobility, greater muscle strength and balance and better coordination.

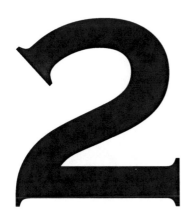

When the Body Breaks Down

Every job has its own set of hazards. As we discussed in the previous chapter, working at a desk job is no different. Where construction workers are exposed to the hazard of hitting their thumb with a hammer and truck drivers are exposed to the risk of suffering from a collision, those of us who work at a desk are exposed to the hazard of developing the Desk Distortion Posture. If you recall, the Desk Distortion Posture involves a specific pattern of abnormal posture, restricted movement, muscle strength imbalance and incoordination.

In this chapter we will explore a number of common physical complaints that are frequently caused by working at a desk, such as headaches, low back pain, neck and upper back pain, wrist and hand pain and leg pain. For each of these complaints, you will learn what causes them as well as simple things that you can do to alleviate their discomfort. All of the exercises and stretches that we will talk about in this chapter will be explained in detail in Chapter 5.

It is important to remember that there are a number of conditions that can cause pain; many of them are no big deal, but some are serious. For this reason, it is important to see your chiropractor if you have pain on a regular basis so he or she can rule out a more sinister condition.

Headaches

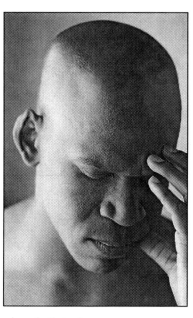

Although headaches can be due to a wide variety of causes, such as drug reactions, temporomandibular joint dysfunction (TMJ), tightness in the neck muscles, low blood sugar, high blood pressure, stress and fatigue, the majority of recurrent headaches are of two types: migraine (vascular) and cervicogenic (muscular). Migraine headaches are called vascular headaches because the pain itself is caused by a dilation of the blood vessels inside the head. Migraine headaches tend to be pounding headaches and are often associated with nausea, sensitivity to light or sound and visual disturbances.

The most common type of headache is what's called the cervicogenic, or tension headache. The word cervicogenic simply means 'beginning (genesis) in the neck (cervico).' There is a small muscle located between the base of the skull and the first vertebrae in the upper neck called the rectus capitis posterior minor (RCPM) muscle. This muscle has a small tendon which slips between the upper neck and the base of the skull to attach to the dura mater – a skin-like tissue that covers that brain. Although the brain itself has no feeling, the dura mater is a very pain-sensitive tissue. Consequently, when the RCPM muscle goes into spasm and its tendon tugs at the dura mater, a headache results.

This single-most important thing you can do to combat cervicogenic headaches is to have routine chiropractic adjustments of the upper neck. Working at a desk job encourages your head to be carried too far forward, placing undue stress at the top of the neck and often causing headaches.

The following Deskercises are the most effective to help avoid headaches at work: the Opening Stretch, the Chair Neck Stretch, the Dumbbell Row and Neck Rolls. It is also helpful to maintain proper head posture by tucking your chin slightly and pushing your head back a couple of inches as illustrated in the Wall Posture exercise.

Low Back Pain

Low back pain is the number one cause of pain and disability in the workplace. There are two primary reasons why workers experience back pain: overuse and disuse. Overuse back pain is the kind of pain you experience when you shovel the snow from your walkway or manually pull weeds in your 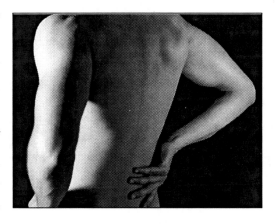 garden. In its mildest form, this type of back pain subsides after a day or two of rest and may not be an indication of bigger problems. However, if you do a lot of bending, lifting or twisting at work and you experience back pain, you may be suffering from an overuse syndrome in the low back. If the cause of the overuse is not corrected, it can lead to injury or permanent disability.

Just as overuse of the low back can cause pain, so can lack of use. It comes as a great surprise to many that sitting is stressful on the low back; at least sitting for extended periods of time. While the stress associated with disuse is less intense than overuse, it can lead to just as much pain and disability. When you sit, your pelvis rolls backward, causing your low back to flatten, your psoas muscles to tighten and your abdominal muscles to become weak. Then when you stand back up again, your low back gets pulled forward by the tight psoas muscles. Since your abdominal muscles are weakened, they don't have the strength to properly support your back. Consequently, your low back becomes much more susceptible to chronic pain and injury.

The best thing that you can do if you are suffering from low back pain is to visit your chiropractor. Chiropractic care has been demonstrated over and over again to be the most effective treatment for low back pain. In addition, there are a number of Deskercises that you can do while you are working which will help to protect and stabilize the low back. The most important are Pelvic Tilts and Chair Crunches to strengthen the abdominals, the Psoas Stretch to decrease tension and Stiff-Leg Deadlifts to strengthen the low back.

Neck and Upper Back Pain

Because working at a desk job requires you to do most of your work with your arms held in front of you, there is a tendency for your shoulders to roll forward, your head to jut forward and for you to lose muscle strength in your mid-back. These three components of the Desk

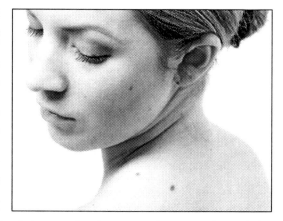

Distortion Posture result in chronic tightness in the trapezius muscles of the upper back, as well as a number of other muscles of the upper back and neck.

Chronically tight muscles in the upper back and neck frequently leads

to some of the joints in the upper spine to become 'stuck.' When these joints become stuck, the area around them becomes swollen and tender to the touch. This chronic tightness and swelling causes irritation of the nerves which run through the area. In addition to pain, this nerve irritation can have a negative impact on the strength of your muscles and even the function of your internal organs. This is one of the reasons why indigestion and stomach ulcers are so common in people who work at desk jobs.

In order to achieve the goal of reducing or eliminating upper back and neck pain, it is necessary to re-establish normal posture. To do this it is necessary to correct four things: loss of joint mobility in the mid-back and neck, weakness in the mid-back muscles, tightness in the upper chest muscles and poor posture in the upper back and neck.

Whenever you are dealing with problems in the neuromusculoskeletal system, chiropractic care is an important first step. Chiropractic is a very effective way to re-establish normal joint motion. The most important Deskercises for the neck and upper back are the Dumbbell Row, the Chair Neck Stretch, the Dumbbell Shrug and the Stick-Em Up Stretch.

Wrist and Hand Pain

Most people who work at desk jobs have to do a lot of work with their hands by typing or writing. Consequently, the additional stress on the hands, wrists and arms when they are not positioned correctly, or when they lose normal flexibility and muscle balance, can lead to a

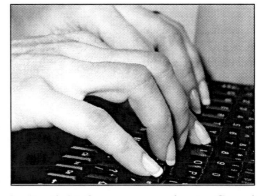

host of problems ranging from chronically tight forearm muscles to Carpal

Tunnel Syndrome.

Carpal Tunnel Syndrome is characterized by pain, numbness or weakness in the hands, caused by the compression of a nerve called the median nerve, which runs through an area of the wrist called the carpal tunnel. The carpal tunnel can become inflamed and swollen if the wrists are not held in the proper position while you work, if the bones in your wrist are not positioned properly or if you overwork your hands without a break. The swelling in the carpal tunnel puts pressure on the median nerve, resulting in pain and weakness in the hands or wrists. If the pain and numbness is primarily in your hands and becomes worse when you have to write or use a keyboard or if the pain in your hands wakes you up at night, you may be suffering from Carpal Tunnel Syndrome and should seek chiropractic care.

Another common cause of wrist and hand pain is simply from using them too much and not taking the time to keep the muscles strong and flexible. Although tight and over-stressed muscles usually lead to pain primarily in the wrists and forearms, pain can sometimes be felt in the hands as well.

In either case, there are a number of Deskercises and stretches which should help, such as the Wrist Stretch and the Prayer Stretch.

Leg Pain

Leg pain can be caused by one of three things: a pinched or irritated nerve, muscle spasm or poor circulation. Most people have heard the term 'sciatica' before. Sciatica is an irritation of the sciatic nerve - a large nerve that comes out of the low back and travels down the leg. If you have pain that 'radiates' or 'shoots' down your leg, it is likely due to the sciatic nerve being pinched or irritated in some way. The irritation of the sciatic nerve is frequently caused by the spasm of a small muscle in the buttock called the piriformis

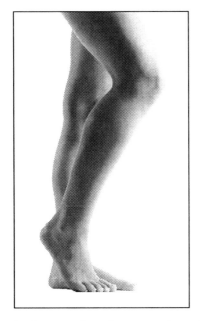

muscle, but it can also be caused from a disc bulge or joint problems in the low back. There is no question that anyone who is experiencing radiating or shooting pains down their leg should seek chiropractic care right away. This type of pain should not be taken lightly.

Chronic tightness in the back of the legs is very common in people who work at desk jobs. This happens because those who have desk jobs typically sit with their knees bent for most of the day. When the knees are bent, the hamstring muscles become shortened and tight. This tension in the hamstrings is not only uncomfortable, but it also restricts the normal motion in the hips and pelvis and increases the tension in the low back.

Another problem that tight leg muscles can cause is a decrease in normal circulation. The muscles in the legs are designed to assist the heart by pumping blood back toward the heart everytime the muscles contract. Without this pumping action of the leg muscles, blood tends to pool in the legs and can contribute to the formation of varicose veins. When the muscles in the legs are chronically tight, they will actually work against proper blood circulation in your legs.

There are a number of Deskercises and stretches that can do wonders to decrease the muscle tension in your legs, decrease the pressure on the sciatic nerve and improve the circulation in your legs. The most important of these are the Triangle Stretch, the Quadriceps Stretch, the Glute Medius Stretch and the Lunge.

So What Do You Do?

If you suffer from headaches, low back pain, neck pain or regular bouts of pain in any other part of your body, there are two things that you need to do. The first is to minimize the stress on your body by organizing your workspace to better accommodate your particular physique. The adjustment of your chair, the height of your computer screen and even the placement of heating and cooling vents can have a tremendous impact on the stress your body has to endure throughout the day. In the next chapter we will discuss how to adjust and organize your workspace to minimize the stress on your body.

The second is to perform specific exercises and stretches which will help to re-establish proper posture, muscle balance, mobility and coordination. The exercises and stretches are described in Chapter 5. But first, let's take a look at ways to minimize the stress on your body when you are at work.

3 Reducing Stress at Your Desk

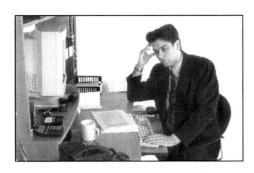

Before getting into the exercises and stretches in the Deskercise program, it's important to look at ways that you can decrease the stress on your body while at work. If you are experiencing discomfort, part of the problem is likely that your workspace is not arranged or adjusted correctly for your body. It may be as simple as just changing the adjustment of your chair, improving your office lighting or re-arranging your work surface.

In this chapter, you will learn how to adjust your chair, set up your computer, and organize your workspace in such a way as to minimize the stress on your body. In addition, we will talk about a number of hidden stressors you may not have thought about, such as poor lighting, drafts and noise that can have an impact on how you feel at work. The more you can reduce or eliminate these sources of stress on your body, the greater the benefit will be from the exercises and stretches and the better you will feel overall.

Fitting Your Chair

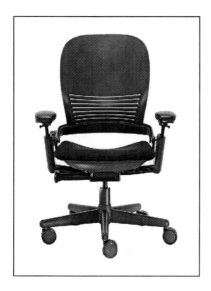

The longer you sit at work each day, the more critical it becomes to have a chair that is properly fitted for your body. If your chair is not adjusted correctly, it forces you into an unhealthy posture; placing a great deal of stress on your muscles and bones and making it difficult to remain comfortable or concentrate on what you are doing. Over time, an improperly adjusted chair can lead to headaches or pain in the arms, upper back, low back or neck. Keeping your chair adjusted correctly is simple and, as long as you are the only one sitting in it, should only have to be checked on occasion.

The correct way to adjust your chair will depend somewhat on the type of work you do and the height of your work surface. In all cases, the goal of properly adjusting your chair is to maintain the curve in your low back and to minimize the stress on your upper back, shoulders and arms. To accomplish this, it is important that your chair be adjusted to have the correct seat angle, the correct lumbar support, the correct height and the correct foot support and arm rests.

The Seat Angle

The first adjustment to properly fit your chair is to set the angle of your seat. Contrary to popular belief, it is not optimal to sit straight up with your hips and knees bent at a 90° angle. This position tends to flatten the low back pretty quickly and leads to stress on the whole body, so you will want to experiment with either tipping the angle of your seat backward slightly or forward slightly to find what is most comfortable for you.

People who do a lot of keying on a computer keyboard or a typewriter often find it most comfortable to tilt the seat back slightly, allowing the body to lean back slightly. It is important that if you angle your seat back, you don't tilt it so much that the front edge of the seat puts pressure on the back of your legs. Tilting your seat backwards slightly allows your low back to maintain its proper curve by resting firmly against the lumbar support.

If your job requires you to do more reading or writing at your desk, you may find it better to tilt the seat forward by ten or fifteen degrees. Tilting the seat forward encourages your pelvis to tip forward, helping you to retain the natural curve in your lumbar spine.

The Lumbar Support

The sole function of the lumbar support on your chair is to encourage the natural curve of your lower spine and to help support your low back muscles by transferring some of the weight of the upper body into the cushion, thereby reducing the load on your low back. In order for this to happen, the seat back should be adjusted up or down so that the curve fits the natural curve of your low back. If it is positioned too low, it will not be able to support your spine properly.

Chair Height

The height of your chair will depend on your height and the height of your work surface. A good place to start is by adjusting your chair so that your elbows are at the same level, or slightly above, your work surface. Ideally, to minimize the stress on your arms, wrists and even your upper back your elbows should be bent between a 90° - 110° angle when you are working.

Foot Support

If your chair must be set high enough so that your feet do not rest comfortably on the floor without the front edge of the seat putting pressure on the back of your legs, it will be important to use a foot rest at your workstation. Ideally, a foot rest should be high enough so that you can slide your hand between the front edge of your seat and the back of your thighs. A good foot rest should also be angled so that your feet are roughly at a natural 90° to your legs so that you don't experience any additional stress to your lower legs.

Arm Rests

The purpose of the arm rests is to decrease the stress on the neck and upper back by supporting some of the weight of the arms. If your chair is equipped with arm rests, they should be adjusted so that they lightly support your forearms when you are working at your usual activity. If they are not set high enough to support your arms while you work, your upper back and neck will suffer additional stress. It is equally important that your arm rests not be set too high. If they are, you will have to hold your shoulders in a raised position in order to work, which also places undue stress on the muscles of your upper back and neck.

Organizing Your Workspace

If you are like most people, you have a variety of items in your workspace, such as a phone, a computer monitor and keyboard, pictures, manuals, forms, a calendar and the like. How these items are arranged can make a significant difference in the amount of stress your body experiences while you are working. In general, your work area should be organized to maximize the amount of time you spend performing tasks which are closest to the Structural Center of your body and to minimize the amount of time you spend performing tasks

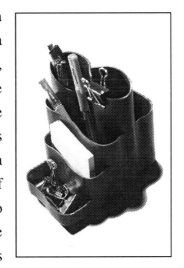

which are furthest away from your body. For simplicity's sake, you may arrange your work space into three areas: the Frequent Use Area, the Occasional Use Area and the Non-Use Area.

Frequent Use Area

This is the area that is closest to your body when you are seated at your desk; covering the area from the front edge of your work surface extending to the end of your finger tips when your elbows are bent 90°. If your job requires that you do most of your work on a computer, this is the area where your keyboard and mouse should be located. If most of your job involves writing, this is where your writing should take place. Whenever possible, you will want to do your work in this area to minimize stress on the body.

Occasional Use Area

The Occasional Use Area extends from the outer edge of the Frequent Use Area to the tips of your fingers when your arms are extended. This is where you should keep items which you use throughout the day, but that you are not currently using. When these items are needed, you simply move them into your Frequent Use Area until you are done with them, at which point you move them back into the Occasional Use Area. Most people find it comfortable for the screen of their monitor to lie somewhere within this area.

Non-Use Area

The Non-Use Area should be reserved for items which you rarely or never need to perform your job. Examples of Non-Use items are pictures of your family, a clock, a business card holder, phone books and the like. Because the demands of jobs vary considerably, as does each individual's physical build, it will be necessary to try different arrangements in order to discover what works the best for you.

Setting Up Your Computer

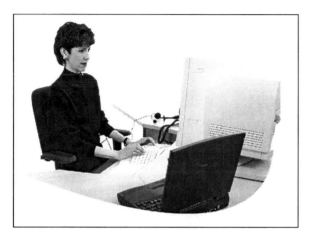

How your computer should be set up in order to minimize the stress on your upper body, wrists and eyes will depend on what kind of work you do. If your work primarily requires you to read and enter data directly from your computer monitor, you should set up your computer so that your monitor is directly in front of you. If you primarily enter information into your computer by reading paper copy, only using your monitor to check your work, you should set the copy in front of you and your computer monitor to either side.

The distance between the computer monitor and your eyes will also depend on the type and the detail of the work you do. You will want to set up your monitor as far away as you can, while keeping it close enough to see what you are doing without eye strain or having to lean your head or body forward. Typically a 24" - 30" range, or about arm's length, works well for most people.

The height of the monitor should be adjusted so that the center of the screen falls somewhere between the bottom of your chin to the top of your chest. If your monitor is higher or lower than that, it may lead to increased stress on your neck.

Your computer keyboard should be kept in your Frequent Use Area unless your primary job requires you to write down information displayed on the computer monitor with only occasional use of the keyboard. In this case, your keyboard could be moved just to the side of your Frequent Use Area.

Whenever possible, the body of the computer itself - the CPU - should be kept outside of the workspace area, unless it is used to prop up your monitor.

Lifting Correctly

There is no single lifting technique that will work in every situation. Lifting a small heavy box off of the floor requires a very different technique than lifting a canoe up onto the roof of your van. For this reason, it's better to learn the six basic rules for safe lifting: keep the load in front of you, minimize bending at the waist, keep the load close to your body, take a wide stance, wear a lumbar support belt and get help with large items. Let's take a look at

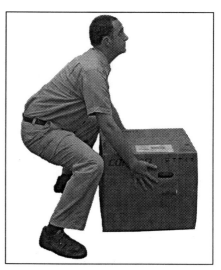

each one of these rules and why they are important for reducing your risk of low back injury.

Rule #1
Keep the Load in Front of You

The bones and muscles of the body have their maximum strength in the center of the body and are weaker and more prone to injury on the sides. This is why you should never twist when you are lifting. When you twist, you rapidly shift the load from the stronger, more resilient muscles, to the weaker, more fragile muscles, dramatically increasing your risk of injury.

Rule #2
Minimize Bending at the Waist

The low back is a very mobile area of the body. Unfortunately, this degree of mobility also makes it more unstable and susceptible to injury than most other parts of the body. Frequent bending at the waist is a very common cause of low back injury because bending at the waist places all of the stress from the weight of your upper body as well as the weight of the item you are lifting directly onto the unstable low back. To reduce the risk of low back injury, you will want to minimize the amount of bending you have to do when lifting. This can be accomplished by bending more at the knees when you have to lift something off the floor and, whenever possible, to position the load at waist-level before lifting it.

Rule #3
Keep the Load Close to Your Body

The closer that you can keep the load to your Structural Center, the less strain it will be on your body. In Chapter 1 you read about women in many parts of the world who are able to carry large pots of water on their heads with very little effort. They can do this simply by keeping the load as close to their Structural Center as possible.

Rule #4
Take a Wide Stance

By taking a wide stance when you have to lift something, it is easier to keep the load closer to your Structural Center, thereby minimizing the stress on your back. It minimizes the amount of bending at the waist by allowing you to keep your hips under your body and it allows you to use the strong muslces of the legs and buttocks to help you lift, rather than the weaker muscles of the low back.

Rule #5
Wear a Lumbar Support Belt

When you lift something heavy, there is an increase in the pressure inside your abdomen. This increase in pressure helps to stablize the low back. To illustrate how this works, think about how a balloon becomes more rigid when you increase the air pressure inside. When the balloon is not filled, it is very floppy and pliable. But, when you increase the pressure on the inside by blowing it up, the balloon becomes rigid. The same happens inside your body. When your abdminals and low back are relaxed, they are very pliable and flexible. But when you lift something heavy, your abdominal muscles contract to increase the pressure inside your belly, thereby making the whole region more rigid and stable.

What does this have to do with a lumbar support belt? The purpose of the lumbar belt is to improve low back stability by supporting the abdominal muscles and increasing the internal pressure of abdomen. The weaker your admoninal muscles are, the more a lumbar support belt will help.

Rule #6
Get Help With Large Items

Every year, many people are injured when they attempt to lift too much. The object that they try to lift may not be too heavy, it may just be too large. A large light-weight box can put as much stress on the back as a small heavy box. Ask someone to help you with heavy or awkward items.

Dodging The Draft

Another source of physical stress at your workstation can occur if your workspace is located next to a drafty window or under a heating or air conditioning vent. When air blows against your neck and upper back, it causes your muscles to tighten up. It is very common for people who have to work in drafty locations to suffer chronic muscle tightness in the neck and upper back and to suffer from headaches just due to the air blowing on their body.

Correcting this problem can be as easy as diverting the air blowing from a vent or keeping an open window closed. If this cannot be done and the air flow bothers you, you should request that your workspace be moved to a more comfortable location.

Quieting the Noise

The constant bustling din of activity present in most work environments is a commonly overlooked source of stress in the workplace. The louder this noise becomes, the greater the stress. Noisy environments make concentrating more difficult, cause the muscles of the upper body to tense up and can lead to headaches, increased susceptibility to illness and fatigue. Common sources of noise are telephones, computer equipment, background music, co-workers' conversations and machinery.

Try sitting at your desk for a few moments with your eyes closed and concentrate on all of the sounds that surround you. Do this several times per day. You may be surprised by how much noise is going on around you, and although you have probably learned to tune it out, excess noise is still a source of stress. If your workplace is noisy, you may want to discuss the issue with your management to find a way to reduce it. If it's stressful to you, it is likely stressful to others. Sometimes something as simple as just turning down the background music or turning down the ringers on the phones will be enough. If this is not possible, it may be necessary to relocate your workspace to a quieter area or to have acoustical panels installed.

Taking a Breather

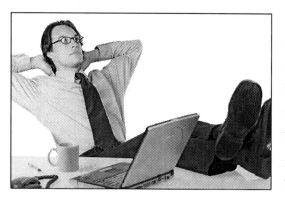

Your body will feel much better throughout your day if you can take several one-minute mini-breaks where you can sit back and take some deep breaths. To do the breathing mini-break, just sit back in your chair, close your eyes and breathe as deeply and as slowly as you can and count to 60. Once you finish your mini-break, you can resume your work refreshed and ready to go.

4 The Deskercise Program Basics

Before we begin describing the individual exercises and stretches of the Deskercise program, it important to understand how to exercise and stretch properly so that you can enjoy their maximum benefits. In this section you will learn what you need to know to exercise and stretch in a safe and effective way.

How to Stretch Properly

Stretching not only feels great, it is also very effective at reducing muscle tension, decreasing stress and maintaining flexibility and joint mobility. In order to experience the benefits of stretching, however, it is important that you stretch correctly. Stretching your muscles too hard, bouncing while holding a stretch or stretching your muscles when they are too cold can lead to muscle injury and a worsening, rather than improvement, in flexibility and muscle tightness. Proper stretching technique is easy, provided you follow a few simple rules.

The first rule is to never stretch your muscles too hard. You should only

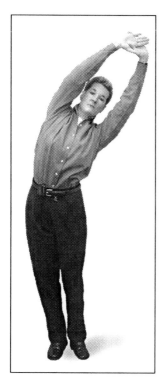

stretch to the point where you can feel a mild pull on the muscle. If you attempt to stretch further, you may cause small muscle tears and a reflex tightening of the muscle. When this happens, it can lead to muscle scarring and counteract the benefits that stretching provides.

The second rule is to never bounce while stretching. When you bounce, you momentarily force your muscles to stretch further than they should, resulting in the same overstretching effects just mentioned.

The third rule is to only stretch your muscles when they are warmed up. Years ago, it was taught that you should stretch before you exercise, but recent research has found that you should stretch only after your muscles have been fully warmed up. Muscles are a lot like plastic. If you heat plastic, you can bend it and stretch it without it breaking. However, if you try to bend or stretch the same piece of plastic when it is cold, it will break. When your muscles are warm, they can be stretched without undue strain. But if you try to stretch your muscles when they are cold, you can injure them by causing small tears in the muscle tissue. For this reason, it is important to stretch your muscles only after you have warmed them up with some exercise and not right after you wake up in the morning.

If you follow these three simple rules - gentle stretching, not bouncing and warming up your muscles before stretching - you will maximize the effectiveness of your stretching routine while minimizing the chances of injuring your muscles.

How to Exercise Correctly

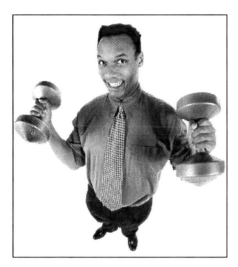

There are two types of exercises that we will be focusing on in this book. The first type is strength exercise. Exercises designed to increase strength are especially useful to improve posture, muscle balance and, of course, strength. In order for your muscles to become stronger, they need to be worked hard enough so that they are slightly overloaded. This is called the "Overload Principle." The Overload Principle simply states that muscles develop strength in direct relation to the demand placed on them. If you place a lot of demand on your muscles through exercise, your muscles will get stronger. However, if your muscles are not exercised enough, they will become weaker.

The biggest mistake that most people make when they begin an exercise program is to underestimate the strength of their muscles. I have had more than one patient tell me that they work out with weights to increase their strength, only to find out that they use very light weights. Building muscle may require heavier weights than you are used to, but you don't need to worry as long as you follow this rule: When you are lifting weights to build muscle, you need the weight to be heavy enough so that you cannot lift the weight more than 15 times. But, the weight needs to be light enough so that you can lift it at least ten times. If you cannot lift it ten times no matter how hard you try, the weight is too heavy. If you can lift it more than 15 times, it is too light.

As you workout and become stronger, the weight that seemed very heavy at first will seem lighter and you will be able to do more repetitions. Once you can reach 15 repetitions, it is time to move to a heavier weight.

The second type of exercise is designed to help you develop endurance and coordination. These exercises, such as walking, climbing stairs and the like, should be done for a longer time than strength-building exercises. The difference between walking for leisure and walking for exercise is the pace. When walking for aerobic exercise, you will want to walk fast enough so that you feel slightly winded - a little short of breath - and maintain that pace for at least 15 minutes. If you can maintain that pace for longer, that is even better. Daily aerobic activity is very important for maintaining good cardiovascular health and weight management and for reducing stress.

What You Will Need

Fortunately, if you work at a desk, you won't need to purchase a lot of equipment in order to keep your body healthy through the Deskercise program. But you will need a few things.

A Desk

A few of the exercises require the use of your desk. Be sure that the surface of your desk will support your body weight prior to doing these exercises. If you have a desk that sits on the floor, this should be no problem. But if your work surface is only attached to the modular walls of a cubicle, you will want to make sure the surface is strong enough. If you have a desk surface that will not support your body weight, a sturdy table in an empty meeting room would work just fine.

A Chair

Any chair will work fine as long as it has arms sturdy enough to support your weight and does not have any wheels. Since virtually all office chairs have wheels, it is important to use a chair other than your office chair for most exercises. After all, you don't want your chair slipping away from you while you are in the middle of an exercise.

A Pair of Dumbbells

Dumbbells are wonderful tools for exercising because of their low cost and their remarkable flexibility. Buy cast dumbbells that are a specific weight rather than dumbbells where you have to add the weights to the handles. The cast dumbbells are safer and easier to manage. I recommend that women start with a pair of 8-pound or 10-pound dumbbells, and men start with a pair of 15-pound or 20-pound dumbbells.

5 Deskercise Stretches And Exercises

If you recall from earlier in the book, the Desk Distortion Posture is a combination of shortened psoas muscles, weakened abdominal and mid-back muscles, shoulders rolled forward, chronic upper back and neck tightness and the head carried forward. The goal of the Deskercise workout is to counteract these effects of working at a desk job and to help you develop better muscle strength, balance, coordination and flexibility. By accomplishing this goal, you will also be improving how you feel physically, improving your work performance and decreasing your stress level. All of the exercises and muscles that will be introduced in the next few paragraphs are covered in detail later in this chapter.

The Basic Deskercise Program

There are five major areas that the Deskercise program is designed to address. These are: weak upper back muscles, tight chest muscles, weak abdominal muscles, tightened psoas muscles and abnormal neck and head posture. Let's start with addressing the issue of weak upper back muscles. When your upper back muscles are weak, your shoulders roll forward, which leads to tightness in your neck and shoulder muscles and contributes to tension headaches. To overcome these symptoms, the primary muscles to strengthen are the rhomboids, which are located in your mid-back between your shoulder blades. Strengthening the rhomboids helps to pull the shoulders back, reducing the stress on the upper back and neck muscles. On the Basic Deskercise Program chart on the next page, you will see an exercise called the Dumbbell Row in the top row. The Dumbbell Row is a very important exercise for strengthening the rhomboid muscles and should be done every day.

On the front side of the upper torso are the muscles of the chest called the pectoralis muscles. One of these muscles in particular, the pectoralis minor, or 'pec minor' muscle, becomes shortened and tight when the shoulders roll forward, as happens when the rhomboids are weak or when you do most of your work out in front of your body. In order to re-establish normal posture in the upper back and neck, it is necessary to stretch out the pec minor muscles using a stretch called the Stick-Em Up Stretch.

The third area to address in most people is weak abdominal muscles. The problem is that when you sit, your abdominal muscles don't get any work. Consequently, they become very weak, very quickly. Weak abdominals cause your pelvis to tip backward, placing added stress on your low back. Strengthening your abdominal muscles is achieved by doing Pelvic Tilts and Power Walking. You will see both of these exercises included in the Basic Deskercise Program chart on the opposite page.

The psoas muscles are very strong, deep muscles that run from your lower spinal vertebrae to the front of your hip. They are the muscles that allow you to lift your knee up in the air when you are standing. When you sit a lot, the psoas muscles become tight. When you stand up again, the tight psoas

The Basic Deskercise Program

Monday	Tuesday	Wednesday	Thursday	Friday
Dumbbell Row	Dumbbell Row	Dumbbell Row	Dumbbell Row	Dumbbell Row
Stick-Em Up Stretch	Stick-Em Up Stretch	Stick-Em Up Stretch	Stick-Em Up Stretch	Stick-Em Up Stretch
Pelvic Tilts	Pelvic Tilts	Pelvic Tilts	Pelvic Tilts	Pelvic Tilts
Psoas Stretch	Psoas Stretch	Psoas Stretch	Psoas Stretch	Psoas Stretch
Wall Posture Exercise	Wall Posture Exercise	Wall Posture Exercise	Wall Posture Exercise	Wall Posture Exercise
Power Walking	Power Walking	Power Walking	Power Walking	Power Walking
Personal Deskercises	Personal Deskercises	Personal Deskercises	Personal Deskercises	Personal Deskercises

muscles pull on your low back resulting in low back pain. Consequently, it is important for anyone who works at a desk job to stretch out their psoas muscles daily.

The fifth major component of the Desk Distortion Posture is the abnormal upper back and neck posture where the head is carried too far forward and the shoulders are rolled forward. Although strengthening the rhomboids will help to address this, it is necessary to train your body to have better posture. This is done with an exercise called the Wall Posture exercise, where you use a wall to check your posture several times a day.

By addressing these five main problem areas, you will make great strides in improving how you feel and your overall neuromusculoskeletal health. In addition to the basic exercises, you may want to include additional exercises for other parts of your body as well. For example, many people find it beneficial to work their triceps to help tighten the back of their arms, or to do additional low back exercises to help stabilize an old injury in their low back. As you go through this chapter, feel free to add any additional exercises that would be beneficial to you or that you would enjoy doing.

In Chapter 7, Doing the Deskercise Program, there are a couple of blank Basic Deskercise Program charts which you can photocopy and complete as you like. One of the tables already has the six exercises of the basic Deskercise program filled in, the other one is completely blank and is for those who want to totally customize their own plan. Whichever you decide to use, I encourage you to have a copy pinned to the wall in your workspace so that you have a daily reminder to do your Deskercises. Now let's take a look at the muscles in the major areas of the body and the exercises and stretches for each.

The Upper Back

The upper back is likely to be the most common area of pain for people who work at desk jobs. To understand why this is, let's review what we learned about the Desk Distortion Posture and how this posture results in the upper back deviating from our Structural Center.

The Structural Center of the body is where all of the weight of your body is supported by your skeleton. When your posture is at your Structural Center, you will experience very little muscle tightness and fatigue because your muscles do not have to constantly work to support you. The physical stresses of working at a desk job force your posture away from this Structural Center, resulting in a predictable pattern of muscle tightness, pain, and decreased flexibility. As described previously, this pattern is called the Desk Distortion Posture and the only way to correct this condition is through specific stretches and exercises.

There are three major muscles which we are concerned about in the upper back: the trapezius, the rhomboid and a big muscle called the latissimus dorsi. There are certainly other muscles in the upper back, but by exercising these three major muscles, problems in the other muscles tend to be minimized.

The trapezius is a very large muscle which runs from the base of the skull to the bottom of the thoracic region of the spine and across to each shoulder. This muscle covers a lot of area. The particular area of this muscle that is a problem for most people is the upper part, which runs between the lower neck, up to the base of the skull and over to the shoulders. This area is often tight, sensitive to the touch and full of trigger points, or 'knots.'

There are three reasons why this happens. The first is that when you suffer from the Desk Distortion Posture your head is carried in front of your Structural Center. So, in order to hold your head up, the trapezius tightens up.

The second reason is that when you suffer from the Desk Distortion Posture, you tend to carry your shoulders higher than they should be. The third reason is that a tight trapezius muscle causes a weakness in your rhomboid muscle, thereby allowing your shoulders to roll forward and up.

The rhomboid muscles attach to the inside edge of the shoulder blade and run across the mid-back to the upper portion of the thoracic spine. The action of the rhomboid muscles is to pull the shoulders down and back and is just about the opposite action of the upper trapezius, which pulls the shoulders up. When the rhomboids are weak and underdeveloped, the tightness in your trapezius will tend to pull your shoulders up, thereby increasing the tension in your upper back and neck. One of the major goals of the Deskercise program is to build up the strength in the rhomboids to restore normal posture and help eliminate the tension in the trapezius.

The latissimus dorsi muscles, also called the 'lat' muscles for short, work with the rhomboids to pull the shoulders down and back. The difference is that the lats attach to the arm, instead of the shoulder blade where the rhomboids attach. For this reason, the lats are also very important to healthy shoulder movement.

Anatomy of the Upper Back

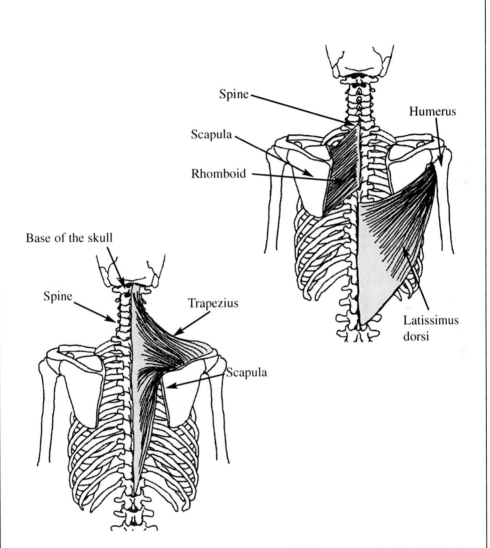

Spine

Humerus

Scapula

Rhomboid

Base of the skull

Spine

Trapezius

Scapula

Latissimus dorsi

The three primary upper back muscles that we will discuss are the rhomboid, the latissimus dorsi and the trapezius. People who have desk jobs will typically suffer from chronic trapezius tightness and soreness, while the rhomboid and latissimus dorsi are usually very weak. This muscular imbalance contributes to neck pain, upper back pain and headaches.

The Dumbbell Row

Benefits: Upper Back Strength

Equipment Needed: Pair of Dumbbells, Chair

Time / Repetitions: 10 - 15 Repetitions

The Dumbbell Row is without question the best overall upper back exercise you can do. It not only develops your rhomboid muscles very well, but it is also a powerful exercise to re-coordinate all of the muscles of the upper and mid-back. It also improves the motion in the entire back and encourages proper posture.

Although this is not a difficult exercise to do, many people find it difficult at first because their upper back muscles are not coordinated. If the Dumbbell Row is done correctly, you should feel the muscles between your shoulder blades getting a good workout. But don't be alarmed if you don't feel anything at first or if you feel it more in your arms. As the muscles in your upper back begin to fire correctly, you should feel the muscles between your shoulder blades working.

To do the Dumbbell Row, place one hand on the seat of your chair and hold a dumbbell in the other. Most people find it comfortable to step back with the outside foot as shown in the picture. Keep your back straight, keep the palm of your dumbbell hand facing toward your legs and allow the dumbbell to hang toward the floor.

Keeping your back straight and your face toward the floor, raise your elbow out to the side and point it toward the ceiling, allowing your upper back to twist so that the dumbbell lightly touches your shoulder. Once the weight has touched your shoulder, gently lower it back down. One repetition should take 4 - 5 seconds.

The Dumbbell Row

Step 1:

Keep your back straight.

Keep your elbow straight.

Step back with your outside leg. This allows your torso to twist easier.

Place your hand on the seat of your chair so that your fingers hang over the front edge.

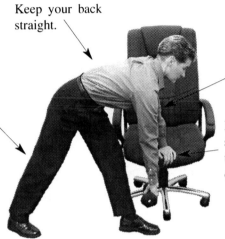

Step 2:

Point your elbow toward the ceiling while lifting the dumbbell up to your shoulder.

Keep your eyes focused on the floor.

Allow your torso to twist so that your chest faces perpendicular to the floor.

Keep your elbow straight.

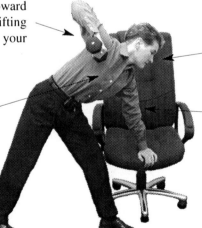

The Dumbbell Shrug

Benefits: Upper Back and Neck Strength

Equipment Needed: Pair of Dumbbells

Time / Repetitions: 10 - 15 Repetitions

The Dumbbell Shrug is a great exercise for the trapezius muscle; especially the upper portion of the muscle which runs from the base of the neck, up to the base of the skull and out to the shoulders. Most people who work at a desk job have a lot of tightness and pain in this area. The Dumbbell Shrug will help to relax the trapezius, increase circulation and decrease the 'knots' in the muscle.

To do the Dumbbell Shrug, stand up straight with a dumbbell in each hand. Draw your shoulders back so that your shoulder blades squeeze together while raising your shoulders as high as you can toward your ears. Then gently let the weights back down again. Each repetition should take 4 - 5 seconds to complete.

The trapezius is considerably stronger than the rhomboid muscle. Consequently, you will be able to lift much more weight doing the Dumbbell Shrug than the Dumbbell Row. However, in order to achieve proper muscle balance in the upper back, I encourage you to use the same weight for both exercises. Here's why: In most people the trapezius is tight, inflamed and full of trigger points and already too strong in comparison to the rhomboid muscle. The goal of exercising the trapezius should not be to make it stronger, but rather to improve blood flow and to decrease the amount of muscle tension. This can be accomplished by exercising the trapezius with a light weight while building strength in the rhomboids.

The Dumbbell Shrug

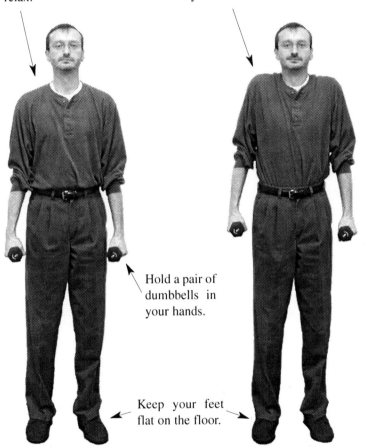

Stand up straight and allow your shoulders to relax.

Draw your shoulders back and up as high as you can. Be sure that your shoulders don't roll forward when you lift.

Hold a pair of dumbbells in your hands.

Keep your feet flat on the floor.

Step 1:

Step 2:

The Opening Stretch

Benefits:	Upper Back and Neck Relaxation
Equipment Needed:	Chair
Time / Repetitions:	30 Seconds

This is a great stretch to help alleviate tension in the upper back and neck. Best of all, it only takes 30 seconds and you don't even have to get out of your chair.

To begin the Opening Stretch, scoot forward in your chair so that you are sitting comfortably on the front portion of your seat. Sit up nice and straight with both feet flat on the floor. With your upper arms hanging down to your side, bend your elbows 90° and turn your palms upward so that they face toward the ceiling.

Now slowly rotate your hands outward, keeping your elbows against your torso, so that you feel a nice squeeze between the shoulder blades. Turn your feet outward as far as you can. Tip your head back slightly to remove the tension from your neck muscles and if you'd like, close your eyes. Take three deep, slow breaths allowing ten seconds for each breath. Just count to yourself as you breathe in "one, two, three, four, five" and back out again "six, seven, eight, nine, ten."

Many people find it beneficial to do this exercise several times during the workday; especially people who do a lot of work on a computer.

The Opening Stretch

Step 1:

Sit up straight and slide to the front edge of your chair.

Bend your elbows 90° and hold them against your side.

Turn your palms upward.

Step 2:

Tilt your head back and take three deep breaths.

Keeping your elbows locked to your side, rotate your hands out as far as you can.

Turn your feet outward.

The Upper Back Stretch

Benefits: Upper Back Flexibility

Equipment Needed: Chair

Time / Repetitions: 15 Seconds on Each Side

The Upper Back Stretch is great for improving the overall mobility and flexibility in your upper back. A very common problem with working at a desk job is that your upper back does not have the opportunity to move very much. Consequently, the joints in your spine get sticky and your muscles shorten. This stretch helps to keep your joints and the muscles in your upper back nice and loose.

To do the Upper Back Stretch, start by sitting up straight in your chair. Take your right hand and place it on the outside of your left knee. Twist your torso toward the left while rounding your upper back until you feel a stretch between your shoulder blades in your upper back as shown on the opposite page. Hold this position for 15 seconds, then do the Upper Back Stretch again to the opposite side.

The Upper Back Stretch

Twist your upper torso while rounding your upper back until you feel a stretch beween your shoulder blades.

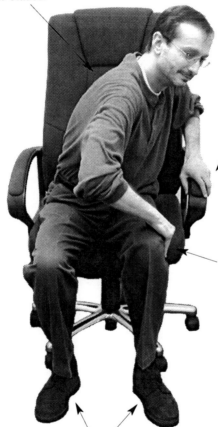

Grip your chair's arm rest with one hand.

Place your other hand on the outside of the opposite knee.

Keep your feet flat on the floor.

The Neck

The ability of the neck is nothing short of amazing. It supports your head, which can weigh up to 16 pounds, and has an incredible range of motion. And it does all of this with only a fraction of the structural support of other areas of the spine. Unfortunately, this degree of movement coupled with limited support results in the neck being especially vulnerable to stress and strain.

In the last section on the upper back we talked about how the Desk Distortion Posture, where the head and the upper back deviate forward from the body's Structural Center, causes muscle spasm and pain in the upper back. Well, the exact same type of muscle spasm occurs in the neck when holding the head forward and allowing the shoulders to roll forward. The muscles that are primarily affected in the neck are the trapezius, the levator scapulae and the scalenes.

As we discussed in the Upper Back section, the trapezius is a very large muscle which runs from the base of the skull, down to the bottom of the thoracic spine. The part of this muscle that is a problem for most people is the upper portion which runs between the base of the neck and the base of the skull. The trapezius muscle is not designed to be the primary muscle responsible for holding up the head. There are a whole host of other neck muscles that are responsible for that task. There are times when those muscles are not strong enough to keep the head up, however, and that is when the trapezius is called in to help. Unlike the normal postural muscles responsible for holding up the head, the trapezius becomes fatigued, tight and sore if it has to help out for very long, which frequently happens in people who work at desk jobs.

The second muscle that we are concerned about is the levator scapulae that runs from the upper inside tip of the shoulder blade to the base of the skull. Like the trapezius, the levator is not designed to help hold up the head for long periods of time. But also like the trapezius, the levator is frequently in a state of continual stress in those who work at desk jobs because of the Desk Distortion Posture.

The third muscle that is of interest to us is actually a group of muscles called the scalene muscles. The scalenes run from the vertebrae in the upper neck down the front of the neck to the upper two ribs. When these muscles become tight, as frequently happens when you work at a desk job, it causes a unique set of problems. There is a bundle of nerves and blood vessels which have to pass around and between the scalenes called the neurovascular bundle. When the scalene muscles become tight, they put pressure on this bundle of nerves and can create the sensation of pain, numbness or tingling in the arms, wrists or hands called Thoracic Outlet Syndrome. Although Thoracic Outlet Syndrome is much more common in women, it can occur in either men or women and should be evaluated by a health care professional such as a chiropractor or neurologist.

The stretches and exercises in this section are designed to improve the posture and muscle tone of all three of these muscles and help alleviate stress, tension or pain in the neck as well as reduce the symptoms of Thoracic Outlet Syndrome.

The Anatomy of the Neck

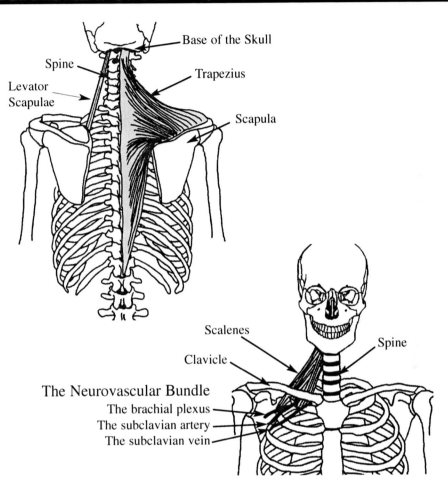

Base of the Skull

Spine

Levator Scapulae

Trapezius

Scapula

Scalenes

Spine

Clavicle

The Neurovascular Bundle
The brachial plexus
The subclavian artery
The subclavian vein

The three muscles of the neck that are the most important to those with desk jobs are the trapezius muscle, which was also discussed in the section on the upper back, the levator scapulae and the scalenes. The scalenes are important because they create a portion of the thoracic outlet, where the nerves and blood vessels that travel down the arm have to squeeze through. When these muscles are tight, it can contribute to pain or tingling in the hands or arms. The trapezius and the levator scapulae create the biggest pain in the neck for most people because these muscles become very tight and painful from poor posture.

Neck Rolls

Benefits:	Neck Mobility
Equipment Needed:	Chair
Time / Repetitions:	15 - 20 Repetitions in Each Direction

This simple exercise is designed to improve mobility in the neck. To do this exercise, scoot up to the front part of your seat and sit up nice and straight. Slowly let your head drop forward and let your chin drop to your chest. From that position slowly rotate your head until your right ear is resting close to your right shoulder. Then, slowly rotate your head back so that your head is tipped back as far as is comfortable. Finally, rotate your head to the left side until your left ear is resting close to your left shoulder.

It is important that you do this exercise slowly and you do not try to force your neck further than it can move comfortably. It is also important to keep your shoulders down while doing Neck Rolls. You can hold the bottom of your seat with both hands if you need help keeping your shoulders down.

Don't be surprised if you hear some crackling in your neck when you perform Neck Rolls. Usually this crackling, also called crepitus, may go away after doing this exercise for a while and poses no hazard. If the crepitus does not go away, it may indicate that there is some scar tissue that has formed in the joint cartilage. Although the crackling may be annoying, it shouldn't be a cause for concern.

If you notice that your neck won't roll as well on one side as it will on the other, there may be some vertebrae that are stuck. This requires chiropractic care in order to help these vertebrae function correctly again.

Neck Rolls

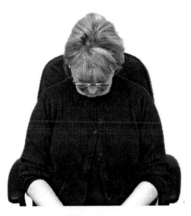

Step 1:

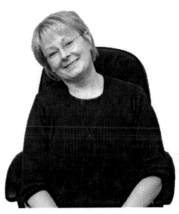

Step 2:

When doing Neck Rolls, it is important to do three things in order to properly stretch the muscles on the neck: 1) keep your shoulders perfectly level, 2) keep your face oriented forward, and 3) roll your head slowly. It should take 30 seconds to make one complete revolution.

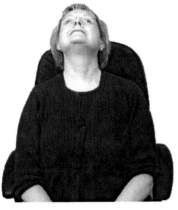

Step 3:

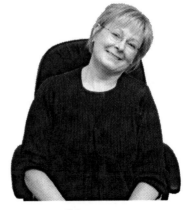

Step 4:

The Chair Neck Stretch

Benefits: Neck Mobility

Equipment Needed: Chair

Time / Repetitions: 30 - 45 Seconds on Each Side

The Chair Neck Stretch can be used to decrease the tightness of the trapezius and levator scapulae as well as the scalene muscles. To do the Chair Neck Stretch, scoot up to the front edge of your chair and sit up straight. With your right hand, grasp the bottom of the seat of your chair. Reach over the top of your head with your left hand and place it on the right side of your head. Gently lean toward the left while tipping your head to the left until you feel a good stretch in the neck and shoulder muscles. Hold this stretch for 30 - 45 seconds, then switch sides.

You can vary the muscles stretched by placing your hand on different parts of your chair seat and leaning your head at different angles. To stretch primarily your trapezius and levator scapulae, grip your seat just behind your hip and tilt your head slightly forward and to the side. To stretch primarily your scalenes, grip your seat at about your mid-thigh and tilt your head slightly backward and to the side. Remember that the muscles of the neck are small and somewhat fragile, so stretch gently and hold without bouncing.

The Chair Neck Stretch

Place your hand on the side of your head and gently pull to increase the stretch on your neck muscles.

Tilt your head to the side until you feel a stretch.

Grip the underside of your seat with one hand.

Place your feet flat on the floor.

The Wall Posture

Benefits: Improved Neck and Upper Back Posture

Equipment Needed: Wall

Time / Repetitions: As Long as Possible

This simple exercise is designed to directly counteract the unhealthy neck and upper back posture found in people who work at desk jobs; namely the head being carried too far forward and hunching of the upper back.

To do this exercise, simply stand up against a wall, making sure that your heels, pelvis, shoulders and the back of your head are all touching the wall. Make sure that your head stays level and that you glide your head backward and that you do not tilt your head back in order to touch the wall with your head. This will require you to pull your chin down toward your chest a bit.

Once you have successfully positioned yourself into this Wall Posture, slowly step away from the wall and go about your business while holding the posture as long as possible. If you have done this correctly, it will probably feel somewhat unusual to walk around like this. But don't worry, you don't look as funny as you feel. As a matter of fact, to everyone else, you probably look better. People with good posture look better than those with bad posture.

It is important that you try to hold this posture while you go back about your business in order to retrain your body mechanics. For this reason, most people find it necessary to do this exercise several times throughout the day as a check-up on their posture.

The Wall Posture

Stand up against a wall so that your shoulders, hips and heels are all touching the wall.

Keeping your head level, draw your neck back until the back of your head touches the wall.

Step away from the wall while maintaining this new head posture. Keep this head posture as long as you can while you work.

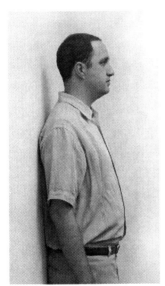

Step 1:

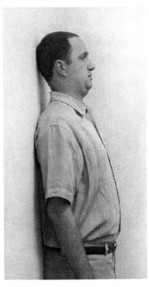

Step 2:

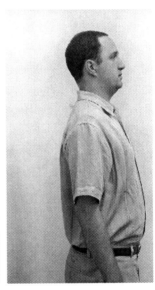

Step 3:

The Low Back and Abdominals

The low back is by far the most frequently injured part of the body. This is due in large part to the fact that the low back, like the neck, is an unstable part of the spine, allowing us to have a lot of mobility, but at the cost of increased risk of injury. Although the low back has much more support from the muscles than the neck does, it is also exposed to dramatically more pressures and stress than the neck.

As long as all of the vertebrae in the lumbar spine are properly aligned and moving correctly and the supporting muscles are healthy and strong, the low back can withstand mind-boggling forces without injury. A professional powerlifter can pick up several hundred pounds off the floor without hurting themselves while performing a deadlift. They are able to do this because of good body mechanics - their bones and joints move correctly, their muscles are strong and coordinated and they maintain good posture.

Those of us who work at a desk job are usually not so lucky. Because most of us sit at our job, sit while we drive to and from work and sit during much of our free time, we lose our healthy body mechanics and become much more prone to pain and injury. The Desk Distortion Posture leaves us with shortened psoas muscles, tight glute medius and piriformis muscles, stressed quadratus lumborum muscles and very weak abdominal muscles. Let's begin with the psoas muscle.

The psoas muscle attaches to the lowest three lumbar vertebrae, runs down through the front of the pelvis and attaches to the upper end of the femur. The psoas is a powerful muscle which allows you to raise your upper leg. When you sit, all of the tension is taken off of the psoas muscle, allowing it to relax. If you sit for many hours every day, the lack of tension of the psoas muscle eventually causes it to shorten. The problem with shortened psoas muscles is that once you straighten your legs and stand up, they pull on the lower lumbar spine, causing back pain.

The glute medius and the piriformis are two muscles in the hip which can also cause problems for people who work at desk jobs. Like the psoas muscle, the glute medius and piriformis lose much of their flexibility and tighten up when you sit for extended periods. This muscle tightness restricts normal motion in the hip joint when you walk, but even more important is the fact that the sciatic nerve, which is the main nerve feeding the leg from the spinal cord, can become entrapped when the piriformis is tight, causing a condition called sciatica. Sciatica is a pattern of shooting pain, numbness or tingling in the leg caused by irritation of the sciatic nerve. The only way to reduce the stress on the sciatic nerve caused by pressure from a tight piriformis muscle is through exercise and stretching.

Although most people don't consider the abdominal muscles to be low back muscles, they actually are one of the most important muscle groups for stabilizing the low back. These also happen to be the least used muscles in people with desk jobs, and consequently they become very weak. The weakened abdominal muscles result in a loss of low back stability and an increased stress on the joints and other muscles, resulting in low back pain. Many people find relief from low back pain simply by exercising and building strength in the abdominal muscles.

The two additional muscles that are a problem for people who work at jobs that require a lot of sitting are the longissimus/erector spinae group and the quadratus lumborum. The difference between these two muscles is that the quadratus lumborum is designed to be an accessory muscle for the low back and is therefore much thinner and weaker than the primary muscles of the low back, the longissimus/erector spinae group. When the low back is not exercised,

Anatomy of the Low Back and Abs

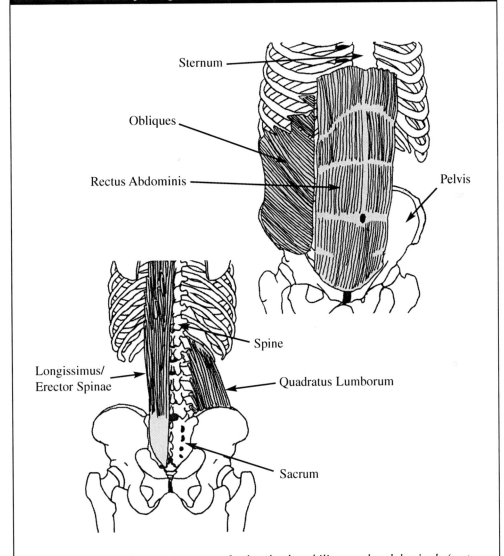

Sternum

Obliques

Rectus Abdominis

Pelvis

Spine

Longissimus/
Erector Spinae

Quadratus Lumborum

Sacrum

The four muscles that are important for low back stability are the abdominals (rectus abdominus), the obliques, the longissimus/erector spinae and the quadratus lumborum. Most people are surprised to find out that strength in the abdominal muscles is critical to low back strength, but it's true. When people sit at a desk for several hours every day, these muscles become weakened, the low back becomes unstable and pain results.

the longissimus/erector spinae group becomes weaker, requiring the quadratus lumborum to pick up some of the slack. Because the quadratus lumborum muscles are not designed to do much lifting, but rather are designed to help rotate and bend the low back, this extra stress causes them to go into spasm and become inflamed.

Problems with shortened and tight psoas and piriformis muscles, weak abdominal and longissimus/erector spinae muscles and stressed quadratus lumborum muscles are very common occurrences in people who have desk jobs. As with the upper body problems associated with the Desk Distortion Posture, the only way to counteract these painful disorders is through the use of exercises and stretches laid out in this book. Let's take a look at the Deskercises for the low back and pelvis.

Anatomy of the Low Back and Abs

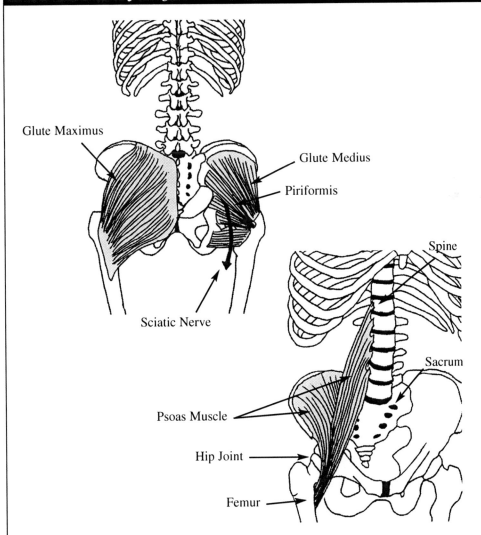

Glute Maximus

Glute Medius

Piriformis

Sciatic Nerve

Spine

Sacrum

Psoas Muscle

Hip Joint

Femur

The three pelvic muscles that are of the most concern to us are the gluteus medius, the piriformis and the psoas (ilio-psoas) muscles. These three muscles are important because when they are tight, they contribute to low back pain and radiating pain in the back of the legs. Due to the angle between the low back and the legs when people sit, these muscles will tighten up quickly and cause pain in people with desk jobs.

Stiff-Leg Deadlifts

Benefits: Low Back Strength and Pelvis Coordination

Equipment Needed: Pair of Dumbbells

Time / Repetitions: 10 - 15 Repetitions

With the exception of abdominal muscle strengthening, the Stiff-Leg Deadlift is the single-most important exercise to strengthen and re-coordinate all of the muscles of the low back and pelvis. To do this exercise, you will want to start by standing up straight with your feet about shoulder-width apart, a pair of dumbbells in your hands and your knees bent slightly - about 10 to 15 degrees. The object is to bend forward at the hips, allowing the dumbbells to drop just below the knees and then to straighten back up again, all the while keeping your head up, your back straight and keeping your knees bent slightly.

It is very important when bending at the hips that you do not cheat and bend at the waist. If you do this exercise correctly, you should feel most of the exercise in your hamstrings rather than in your lower back. If you feel it mostly in your low back, it means that you are not pushing your hips back far enough and that you are bending at the waist. Many people find it helpful to imagine that they are carefully sitting down on a chair behind them while keeping their back straight.

You will want each repetition of lowering the weights down and lifting them back up to take approximately 6-8 seconds. One other thing about the Stiff-Leg Deadlifts: Since you are working large muscles, you will want to use dumbbells that are heavy enough to challenge the muscles. 15 - 25 pound dumbbells are probably a good place to start.

Stiff-Leg Deadlifts

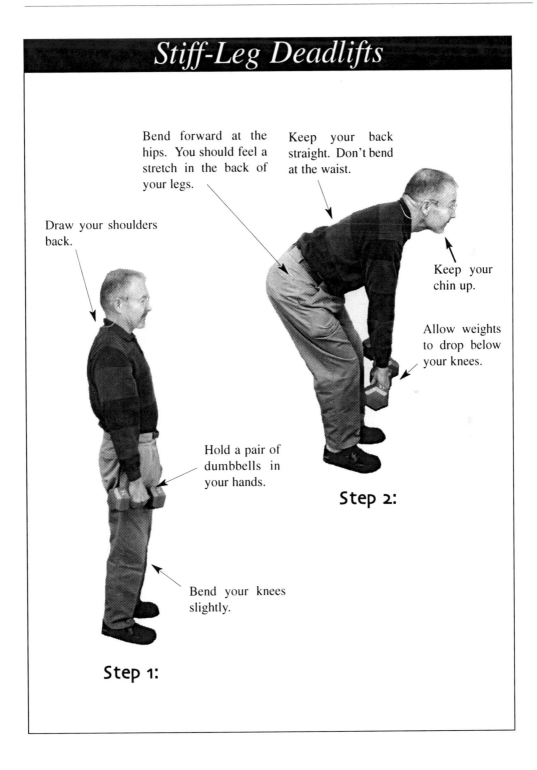

Bend forward at the hips. You should feel a stretch in the back of your legs.

Keep your back straight. Don't bend at the waist.

Draw your shoulders back.

Keep your chin up.

Allow weights to drop below your knees.

Hold a pair of dumbbells in your hands.

Step 2:

Bend your knees slightly.

Step 1:

Pelvic Tilts

Benefits: Abdominal Strength

Equipment Needed: None

Time / Repetitions: As Many as Possible

Pelvic Tilts are one of the easiest exercises to help increase abdominal strength. To do this exercise, stand up straight and place your hands on your hips. Exhale completely while contracting your abdominal muscles and tilting your pelvis as shown in the picture on the opposite page. Hold this position for three seconds, then inhale and allow your body to return to the starting position. Each repetition should take approximately 3 - 4 seconds.

Depending on the condition of your body when you begin doing Pelvic Tilts, you may feel your abdominals getting a good workout from this exercise, but don't be discouraged if you do not feel this at first.

You can make this exercise even more intense by drawing your abdomen in as far as you can after you completely exhale. You should feel a contraction in your oblique muscles just to the side of your abdominals. This extra contraction of the obliques helps to flatten the belly.

Pelvic Tilts

Step 1:

Step 2:

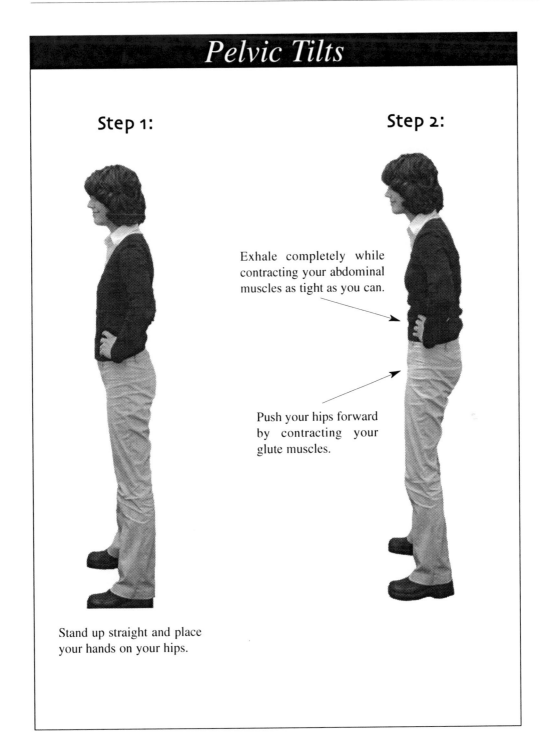

Exhale completely while contracting your abdominal muscles as tight as you can.

Push your hips forward by contracting your glute muscles.

Stand up straight and place your hands on your hips.

Chair Crunches

Benefits: Abdominal Strength

Equipment Needed: Chair

Time / Repetitions: As Many as Possible

Chair Crunches are designed to help increase abdominal strength while improving balance and coordination. To do this exercise, scoot forward in the seat of your chair so that your buttocks rest on the front edge of the seat, but the backs of your legs are not touching the chair. Keeping your back straight, lean back slightly and grip the armrests of your chair with both hands. Using your abdominal muscles, raise your knees as far toward your chest as you can. Hold this position for one second and then slowly lower your knees back down. Each repetition should take approximately 3 - 4 seconds.

You can decrease the difficulty of this exercise by keeping your knees bent so that your feet stay close to your body. The more you straighten your legs, the more difficult this exercise becomes.

Depending on the condition of your body when you begin doing Chair Crunches, you may feel your abdominals getting a good workout from this exercise, but don't be discouraged if you do not feel this at first. Initially, you may feel it more in your low back or even legs. This is common when the abdominal muscles lose their natural coordination. Just keep at it and soon your abdominal muscles will come around.

Chair Crunches

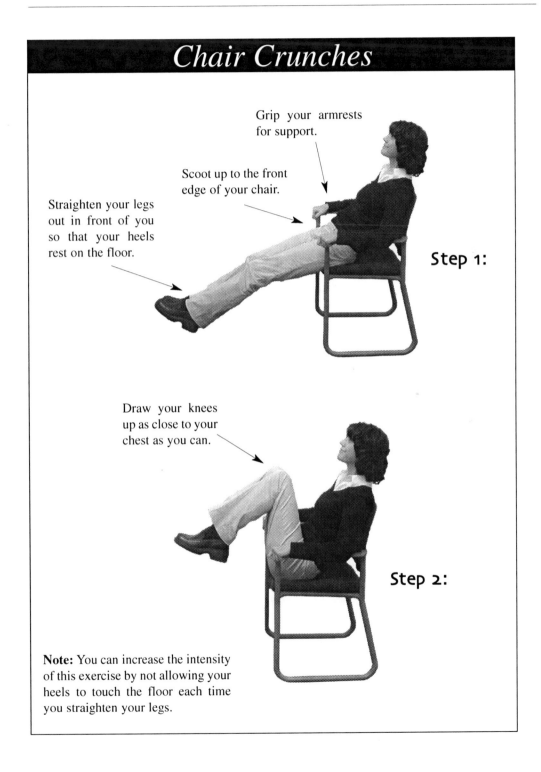

Grip your armrests for support.

Scoot up to the front edge of your chair.

Straighten your legs out in front of you so that your heels rest on the floor.

Step 1:

Draw your knees up as close to your chest as you can.

Step 2:

Note: You can increase the intensity of this exercise by not allowing your heels to touch the floor each time you straighten your legs.

The Cobra Stretch

Benefits: Mobility and Flexibility in the Low Back

Equipment Needed: Chair

Time / Repetitions: 30 - 45 Seconds

The Cobra Stretch is great for improving the flexibility of the abdominal and psoas muscles as well as increasing mobility in the low back. When doing this exercise, be sure that your chair is pushed up against a wall so that it doesn't move away from you. To do the Cobra Stretch, stand facing your chair, with your feet shoulder-width apart and about 24" - 36" away from the edge of your chair. Lean forward and grip the center of your armrests. Keeping your arms straight, allow your pelvis to drop toward the seat of your chair and lift your chin toward the ceiling. You should feel a considerable stretch in the abdominals when you do this stretch correctly.

You can adjust the intensity of the stretch by how far you place your feet from your chair. The further away your feet are, the more intense the stretch will be on your abdominal muscles.

Depending on the strength of your upper body, you may find it difficult to support your weight with your arms for very long. If this happens, you can step forward with your feet slightly to decrease the weight supported by the arms and make sure that you keep your elbows straight. After a few weeks of doing this stretch, your arms will become stronger and it will be easier to support yourself.

Discontinue doing this stretch if you feel pain in your low back, and just stick with the other low back exercises and stretches for a couple of weeks before trying this stretch again. As your back becomes healthier, you should be able to do this stretch without experiencing back pain.

The Cobra Stretch

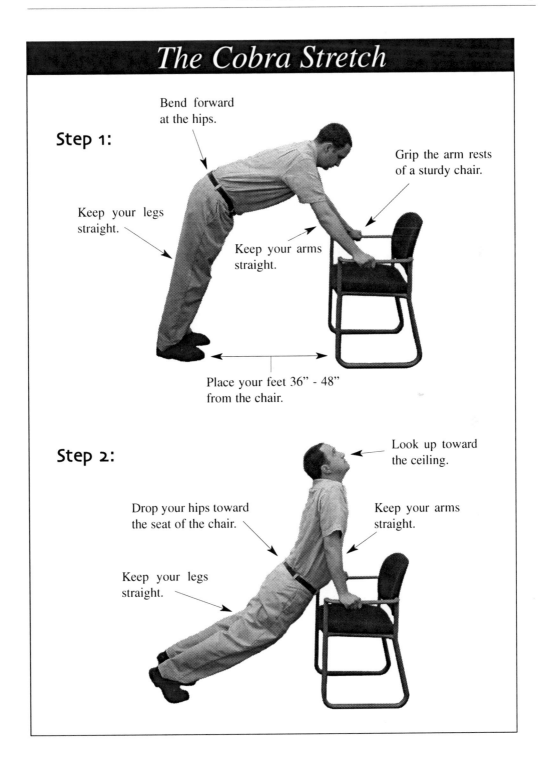

Step 1:

Bend forward at the hips.

Grip the arm rests of a sturdy chair.

Keep your legs straight.

Keep your arms straight.

Place your feet 36" - 48" from the chair.

Step 2:

Look up toward the ceiling.

Drop your hips toward the seat of the chair.

Keep your arms straight.

Keep your legs straight.

The Chair Low Back Stretch

Benefits: Decreased Tension in the Low Back

Equipment Needed: Chair

Time / Repetitions: 30 - 45 Seconds

This stretch is a quick way to reduce tension in the low back and is perfect for a mini-break during the day. To do this stretch, scoot forward to the front part of your seat and straighten your legs. Allowing your spine to bend forward reach your hands as far down the front of your legs as possible and allow your head to drop toward your thighs. Take slow, deep breaths for 30 - 45 seconds, then sit back up again.

If you have a difficult time getting your low back to bend forward, which many people do, it could be for a couple of reasons. The first is that if your hamstring muscles are too tight, they will hold your pelvis in place and not allow it to roll forward. If your pelvis cannot roll forward, your low back will not be able to bend as far forward. If this is the case with you, doing one of the hamstring stretches discussed in the next section will help.

The other reason why you may not be able roll your back forward is that the joints in your low back are stuck and are not allowing the vertebrae to move correctly. This is very common among people who work at desk jobs. The only way to get the joints in the low back moving correctly again is through chiropractic care. If this stretch is difficult for you, it is a good idea to have your low back checked out by a chiropractor.

The Chair Low Back Stretch

Allow your upper back to bend forward.

Bend as much as you can at your hips.

Reach toward your feet.

Scoot up to the front edge of your seat.

Keep your legs straight.

Place your feet flat on the floor.

The Glute Medius Stretch

Benefits:	Pelvis and Hip Flexibility
Equipment Needed:	Chair
Time / Repetitions:	30 - 45 Seconds on Each Side

The Glute Medius Stretch is very effective in reducing the stress in the hip and buttock area. To do this stretch, scoot up to the front part of your seat and rest the ankle of one leg on the thigh of the other. Sit up nice and straight and place both hands around the knee of your topmost leg, interlacing your fingers. Using a gentle pull, draw your knee up to the opposite shoulder and hold the position for 30 - 45 seconds. Then switch legs and do the same stretch to the other leg. If you do this stretch correctly, you should feel a good stretch in the buttock.

This stretch is very important for people who sit a lot at work because the muscles in the buttocks and pelvis become very tight. This tightness contributes to pain and loss of flexibility in the low back.

If you find that you don't have enough flexibility to cross your legs as pictured, you can start by gripping one knee with both of your hands and pulling your knee toward your chest and holding the stretch for 30 - 45 seconds. Over time, the glute medius and piriformis muscles will relax and allow you to perform the stretch as shown.

The Glute Medius Stretch

Step 1:

Sit up straight in your chair.

Cross one leg over the other and grab your knee with both hands.

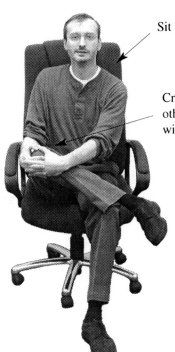

Step 2:

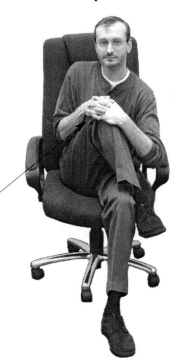

Keeping your back straight, pull your knee up as high up toward the opposite shoulder as you can. Hold stretch for 30-45 seconds.

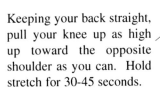

The Psoas Stretch

Benefits:	Low Back and Pelvis Flexibility
Equipment Needed:	None
Time / Repetitions:	30 - 45 Seconds on Each Side

A tight psoas muscle is one of the biggest contributors to the low back pain experienced by most people who sit at work. This stretch is designed to decrease the tension in the psoas muscle and improve the mobility and flexibility in the low back. To do this stretch, start with both feet together, your back straight and one of your hands resting on your chair or a wall for balance. Take a large step back with one of your legs as shown in the picture on the opposite page. Keeping your back leg straight and allowing your front leg to bend at the knee, push the hip of your back leg forward until you feel a stretch in the upper inside front part of the thigh. Hold this stretch for 30 - 45 seconds, then switch legs.

The key to doing this stretch is keeping the hips in the correct position. If you do not feel a stretch in the right place, it is likely that you are allowing your hips to turn to the side and are not keeping them facing the front. The other thing that could be happening is that you may be trying to keep your back foot flat on the floor. In order for the back leg to have enough mobility to stretch the psoas muscle, it will be necessary to raise your heel.

If you have good balance, you can increase the intensity of the stretch by raising your hands above your head and tipping your upper body backwards slightly while looking at the ceiling. This offers you the added benefit of stretching the abdominal muscles at the same time.

The Psoas Stretch

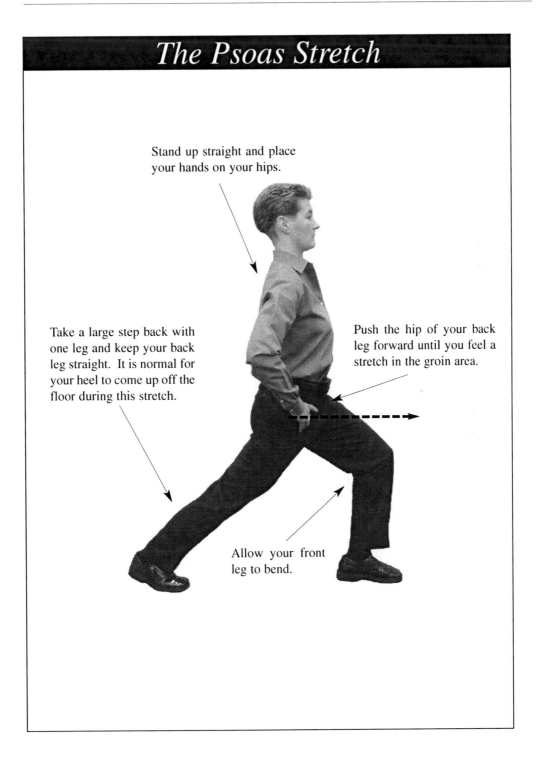

Stand up straight and place your hands on your hips.

Take a large step back with one leg and keep your back leg straight. It is normal for your heel to come up off the floor during this stretch.

Push the hip of your back leg forward until you feel a stretch in the groin area.

Allow your front leg to bend.

The Legs

When you sit for a good portion of your day, the muscles in your legs lose their strength and become tight. Since your leg muscles are responsible for stabilizing your knees, ankles and hips, as well as for moving your body from one place to another, it is important that they be strong, flexible and well coordinated. The major muscle groups that we will address here are the calf muscles, the soleus and the gastrocnemius, and the upper leg muscles, the hamstrings, the adductors and the quadriceps.

The calf muscles are very strong muscles in the back of your lower leg which are responsible for lifting your heel as you walk, allowing you to have a normal walking rhythm. When your calf muscles are tight, the movement in your ankle is restricted, resulting in increased stress on the knees. It is also important for normal blood flow in the legs that these muscles be relaxed, but toned. In addition, tight and deconditioned calf muscles tend to go into painful spasms, especially at night.

The hamstring muscles run from the bottom of the pelvis down the back of your leg and attach to your lower leg bones just below your knee joint. Your hamstrings are responsible for bending your knee and assisting in straightening up your back when you are bent forward at the hips. When you sit for an extended period of time with your knees bent, the hamstring muscles tend to become very tight and to lose strength. Tight hamstring muscles are not only uncomfortable, but they increase stress in the low back by restricting the normal movement of the pelvis, and they increase stress in the knees by restricting normal joint motion.

The adductors are a group of **muscles** which function together to pull your legs toward each other. Because **of the** position of our pelvis and legs when we sit in a chair, these muscles will lose much of their flexibility over time. When these muscles become tight, it results in a loss of normal movement in the hips and pelvis and increases the amount of stress on the low back, hips and knees. The triangle stretch in this section is designed specifically to stretch the adductors as well as the hamstrings.

The other major muscle group of the lower extremity is the quadriceps muscle. This muscle group is actually made up of four individual muscles (hence the name "quad") that work together to straighten your leg. When you sit a lot for a living, your quadriceps muscles become weak. Since this muscle group plays such a major role in the stability of the knee joint, weakness in the quadriceps can contribute to knee instability and pain.

The stretches and exercises in this section are designed to improve the posture and muscle tone of all four of these muscle groups and to reduce the stress, tension or pain in the legs, pelvis and low back.

Anatomy of the Legs

(front view)

(rear view)

Pelvis

Quadriceps

Femur

Hamstrings

Pelvis

Adductors

Fibula

Femur

Tibia

Gastrocnemius

Soleus

Heel

Achilles Tendon

Fibula

The four muscle groups of the legs that we are most concerned about are the calf muscles, hamstrings, adductors and quadriceps. Sitting at a desk for most of the day leads to weakness in the quadriceps and tightness in the hamstrings and adductors. Not only does this cause additional stress on the knees, but also contributes to decreased circulation in the legs and increased pain.

The Lunge

Benefits: Quadriceps and Glute Strength

Equipment Needed: Chair

Time / Repetitions: 10 - 15 Repetitions for Each Leg

You can do Lunges with or without weights depending on your physical condition. If you have not done Lunges before, I suggest that you start without weights. To do the Lunge, start with your feet together and one hand resting on the back of a chair for balance. Step back with one leg so that your legs are about 60° apart. Keeping your back straight, allow your knees to bend until you touch the floor with the knee of your back leg, then straighten your legs again. Repeat this exercise 10 - 15 times for each leg.

If you have knee problems, you may have to modify the Lunge somewhat to make it easier on your knees. One way of doing this is to place a phone book or two on the floor in front of your back leg so that your back knee only drops to within six inches from the floor. If this is still too stressful for your knees, just go down as far as you can. The further down you can go, the better, as long as it doesn't strain your knees.

This is a great exercise to improve the strength and flexibility in the quadriceps and glute muscles as well as to improve your overall coordination and sense of balance. After doing Lunges for a while, you will notice that it is easier to climb stairs, easier to squat down to grab something off of the floor and that there will be less soreness in your buttocks and legs from prolonged sitting.

The Lunge

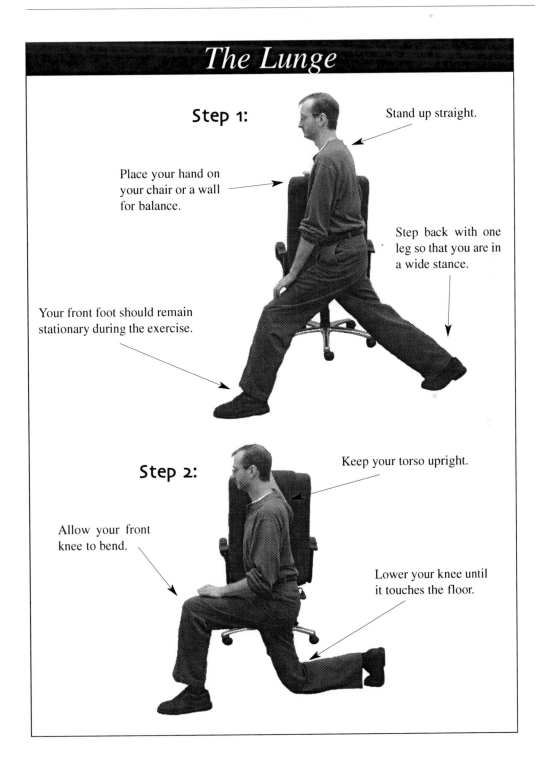

Step 1:

Stand up straight.

Place your hand on your chair or a wall for balance.

Step back with one leg so that you are in a wide stance.

Your front foot should remain stationary during the exercise.

Step 2:

Keep your torso upright.

Allow your front knee to bend.

Lower your knee until it touches the floor.

Calf Raises

Benefits:	Calf Strength
Equipment Needed:	Stair Step or Phone Book
Time / Repetitions:	20 - 30 Repetitions

Calf Raises are great for improving the strength and flexibility of your calf muscles. To do Calf Raises you will need a phone book or a stair step. Begin by placing the ball of your foot on the edge of the step or phone book so that your heel hangs freely in the air. Slowly lower your heel as far as you can, then raise your heel up as high as you can and hold this for one second. You will probably have to place your hand on the back of your chair or on a wall to maintain your balance when doing this exercise. Repeat this exercise 20 - 30 times.

One of the problems with a desk job is that most people begin to suffer the effects from decreased circulation in the legs. The veins in your legs require the exercise of the leg muscles in order to move your blood back to your heart effectively. When this does not happen, you can develop varicose and spider veins as well as swelling around the ankles.

The leg exercises in this section will go a long way to counteracting the decreased circulation in the legs associated with sitting.

Calf Raises

When doing Calf Raises, you will want to place your hand on a chair or a wall to help maintain your balance.

Place the ball of your foot at the edge of the phone book, allowing your heels to hang over the edge.

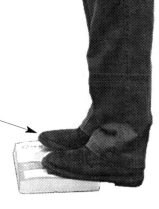

Step 1:

Lift your heels up as high as you can and hold them in this position for one second before lowering them back to the floor.

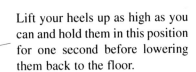

Step 2:

As an alternative, you can do this exercise on a stair step or any other object that is at least 2" high. To make this exercise a bit more challenging, try doing this exercise using only one leg at a time.

The Quadriceps Stretch

Benefits: Quadriceps Flexibility

Equipment Needed: None

Time / Repetitions: 30 - 45 Seconds on Each Side

The Quadriceps Stretch is a great way to reduce the tension and improve the flexibility in the front of the thigh. To do the Quadriceps Stretch start by standing next to chair or a wall and placing your hand on it for balance. Raise one foot backwards by bending your knee and grasping the foot with your free hand. Gently pull your leg back and press your foot against your buttock until you feel a stretch in the front part of your thigh. Hold this position for 30 - 45 seconds, then slowly release your hand from your foot and allow your foot to drop back to the floor. Repeat this stretch on the opposite leg.

Since the quadriceps are such big muscle groups, you will notice an immediate decrease in your overall tension level just by doing this stretch. This maneuver along with the next two stretches for the hamstrings and the calves should be done at least once a day for maximum benefit. I recommend doing each of these stretches twice per day, once early and once in the later part of the day.

The Quadriceps Stretch

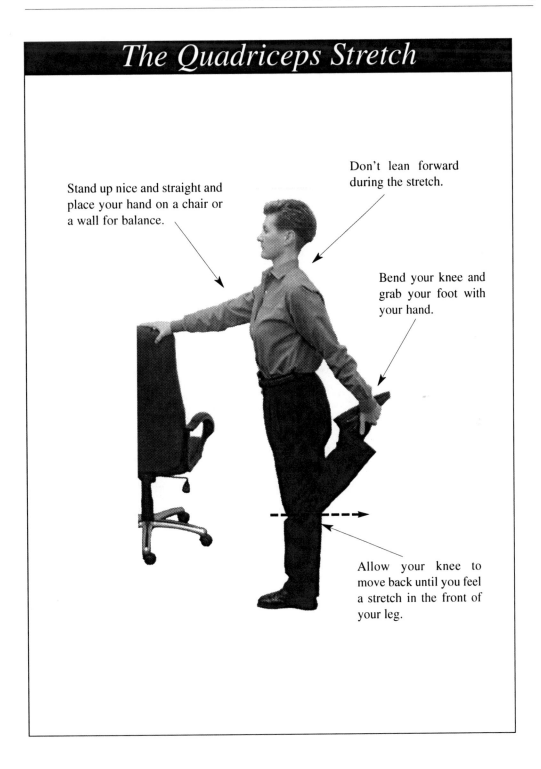

Stand up nice and straight and place your hand on a chair or a wall for balance.

Don't lean forward during the stretch.

Bend your knee and grab your foot with your hand.

Allow your knee to move back until you feel a stretch in the front of your leg.

The Triangle Stretch

Benefits:	Hamstrings and Adductor Flexibility
Equipment Needed:	Chair
Time / Repetitions:	30 - 45 Seconds

The Triangle Stretch is great for improving the flexibility of the hamstrings and adductors. To do this stretch, start by facing your chair, place both hands on the arm rests and place your feet as far apart as you comfortably can. Slowly bend at the hips so that your pelvis drops back behind your feet and your body drops toward the seat of your chair. You should feel a good stretch in your hamstrings, as well as in the inside part of your upper leg. Hold this stretch for 30 - 45 seconds without bouncing.

If you don't feel a stretch in the back of your legs, you may be doing one of three things incorrectly. First, you may have your feet too far away from the chair; try moving your feet a little closer. Second, you may not have your feet spread far enough; try moving them a little farther apart. Third, you may be bending at the waist instead of at the hips; try bending more at the hips as in the Stiff-Leg Deadlifts.

The Triangle Stretch is a must for people with desk jobs as prolonged sitting causes the hamstrings to tighten up. If you do this stretch regularly, you will notice an improvement in your flexibility, you will be more comfortable when you have to sit for long periods and it will even decrease the stress on your low back, helping to reduce back pain.

The Triangle Stretch

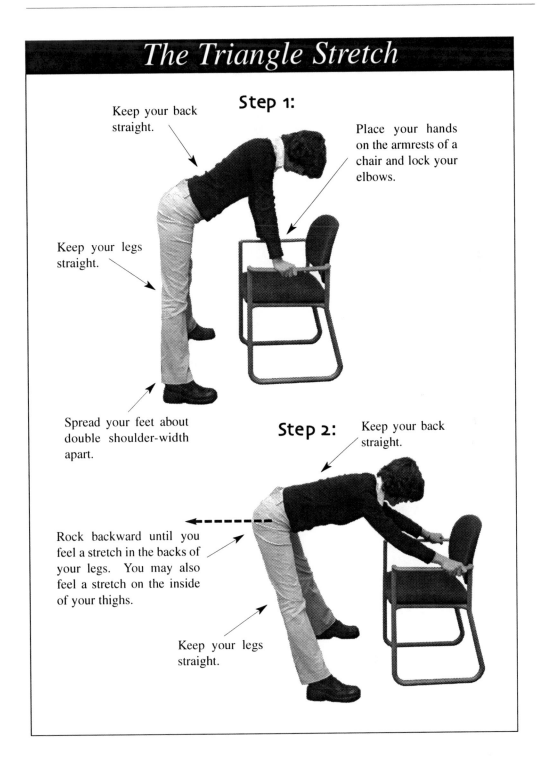

Step 1:

Keep your back straight.

Place your hands on the armrests of a chair and lock your elbows.

Keep your legs straight.

Spread your feet about double shoulder-width apart.

Step 2: Keep your back straight.

Rock backward until you feel a stretch in the backs of your legs. You may also feel a stretch on the inside of your thighs.

Keep your legs straight.

The Calf Stretch

Benefits: Calf Flexibility

Equipment Needed: Wall

Time / Repetitions: 30 - 45 Seconds on Each Side

The Calf Stretch is one of three important stretches, along with the Triangle Stretch and the Quadriceps Stretch, that will keep your legs flexible and relaxed during a long day at work. To do this stretch, start by facing a wall approximately arm's-length away. Place both hands on the wall and take a big step back with one of your legs, allowing the leg closest to the wall to bend at the knee. Gently allow your back heel to drop toward the floor until you feel a stretch in your calf muscles. Hold this stretch for 30 - 45 seconds without bouncing, then switch legs.

As you read in the introduction to this section, the calf muscles are not only responsible for walking, but they also help with pumping blood back to the heart. When the calf muscles, and to some degree the hamstrings, are chronically tight and don't get enough exercise, blood tends to pool in the lower legs and can lead to painful varicose veins and swelling in the ankles.

The Calf Stretch

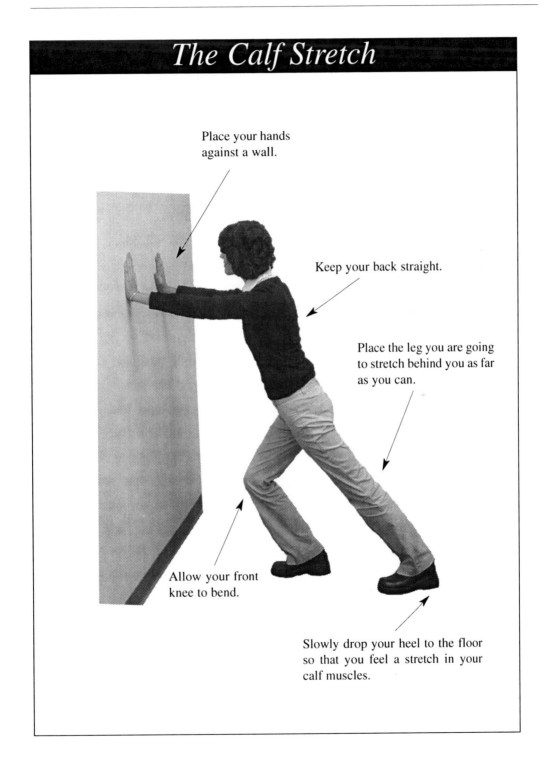

Place your hands against a wall.

Keep your back straight.

Place the leg you are going to stretch behind you as far as you can.

Allow your front knee to bend.

Slowly drop your heel to the floor so that you feel a stretch in your calf muscles.

The Chest

There are two major muscle groups in the chest. These are called the pectoralis major, or simply "pec major," and the pectoralis minor, or "pec minor." In people who work at desk jobs, the pec major muscle tends to become weak from lack of use and the pec minor muscle tends to become tight due to the forward position in which the arms are held.

The pec major muscle is a large muscle group that allows us to push our arms out in front of us. This is the muscle group that is worked when we do push-ups or a bench press. Because the pec major muscle is rarely, if ever, called upon in our daily routine, this muscle usually does not become tight. As a matter of fact, unless we make a point to regularly exercise the pec major muscle it will become weak. You will learn a simple exercise called Desk Push-Ups, which will help to maintain good pec major strength.

The pec minor, unlike the pec major, tends to go into spasm in people who work on computers or any other activity where the arms are held out in front of the body for extended periods. When the pec minor goes into spasm, it can trap and impinge a group of nerves and blood vessels that runs down the arm called the neurovascular bundle. When this group of nerves and vessels are impinged either by tight scalene muscles in the neck or tight pec minor muscles, you may experience cold hands, a tingling sensation or weakness in the arms or hands, especially when your arms are raised over your head - a condition called Thoracic Outlet Syndrome.

In this section you will learn an exercise and a stretch for the chest to keep the pec major strong and to keep the pec minor relaxed and flexible.

Anatomy of the Chest

Clavicle

Pectoralis Major

Humerus

Sternum

Coracoid Process of the Scapula

Pectoralis Minor

The Neurovascular Bundle
The brachial plexus
The subclavian artery
The subclavian vein

3rd, 4th & 5th Ribs

The two primary muscles of the chest, the pectoralis major and minor, are important for not only for upper body strength, but also for allowing the nerves from the neck and the vessels coming from the heart to travel down the arm. If the pectoralis minor muscle is tight, it can put pressure on these vessels and nerves causing pain or tingling into the arms or hands.

Desk Push-Ups

Benefits:	Pec Major Strength
Equipment Needed:	Desk
Time / Repetitions:	10 - 20 Repetitions

Desk Push-Ups are a great way to improve the strength of the pec major muscles. To do this exercise, start by placing both hands on the edge of your desk. Step back so that your body is angled about 45° from the floor and hold your body away from your desk with your arms straight. Bend your elbows and lower your body all the way down until your chest touches the front edge of the desk, then straighten your arms again to raise your body back up. Repeat this exercise for a total of 10 - 20 repetitions.

If you haven't done much strength training, this exercise may seem very difficult or impossible at first. If you are unable to do at least ten push-ups where you touch your chest to your desk, start out by only going down half-way. It is important to do at least ten repetitions in order to work the muscle enough to increase strength. As you become stronger, you will be able to drop your body closer and closer to your desk. One other thing that you can do if you find this exercise too challenging at first is to place your feet closer to your desk. The closer your feet are to your desk, the easier this exercise will be; at least to a point. You can modify this exercise as you need as long as you are able to do the exercise comfortably.

Desk Push-Ups

Keep your back straight.

Place your feet back far enough so that your body makes a 45° angle to the floor.

Place your hands on the edge of your desk.

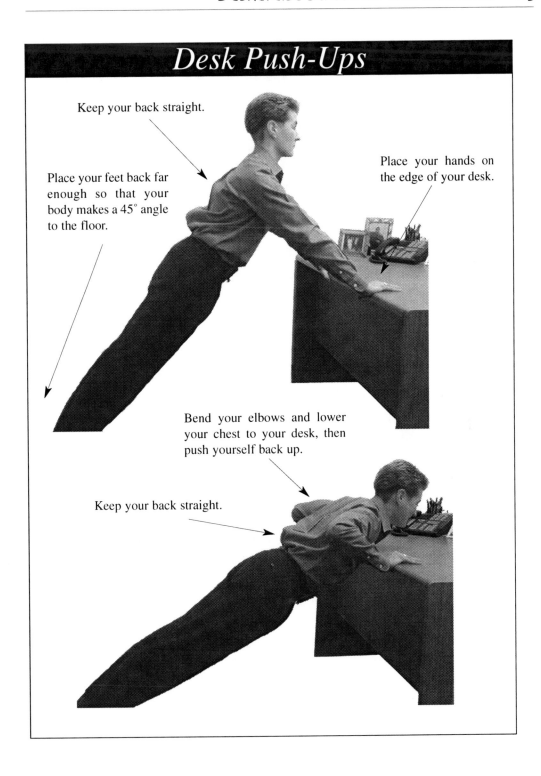

Bend your elbows and lower your chest to your desk, then push yourself back up.

Keep your back straight.

The Stick-Em Up Stretch

Benefits: Pec Minor Flexibility

Equipment Needed: Doorway

Time / Repetitions: 30 - 45 Seconds

The Stick-Em Up Stretch is great for decreasing the tension of the pec minor muscle, allowing the shoulders to roll back to a healthier posture and decreasing any tingling and numbness in the arms that may be present. This stretch is called the Stick-Em Up stretch because you start by assuming the posture often seen in old Western movies when the villain says "Stick'em up!" Your upper arms should be parallel to the floor, with your elbows bent 90° so that your hands are raised above your head with your palms facing forward. With your arms in that position, step into a doorway so that your forearms rest against the door frame. Be sure that your feet are centered within the doorway. Gently push your hips forward until you feel a stretch in your upper chest and shoulders. Hold this position without bouncing for 30 - 45 seconds, then step away from the doorway and allow your hands to drop to your side.

It is important that this stretch be done on a daily basis. When the pec minor is tight, it causes one of the major components of the Desk Distortion Posture - the dreaded forward shoulders as well as the resultant hunching of the upper back.

The Stick-Em Up Stretch

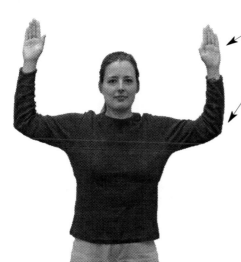

Face your palms forward.

Bend your elbows 90° and raise your upper arms so that they are parallel to the floor.

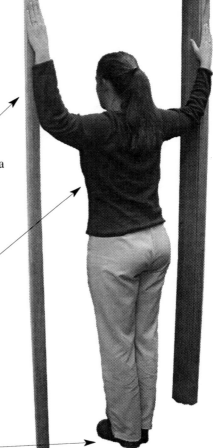

Place your forearms against a door frame.

Stand up straight and gently lean forward until you feel a stretch in your upper pecs. Hold this position for 30-45 seconds.

Bring your feet into the doorway so that you are not bending forward.

The Arms

Keeping the muscles and joints in the arms mobile, flexible, strong and coordinated poses a different set of challenges than in the other parts of the body for the simple reason that those of us who work at desk jobs use our arms, wrists and hands all day long. Unlike the legs where the biggest culprit behind the pain and tightness is the lack of use, the biggest problem with the arms is overuse. For example, the biceps muscle on the front of the upper arm is often chronically tight, the triceps muscle on the back of the upper arm is very weak, the forearm muscles tend to become very tight and ropy and many people develop a condition in their wrists and hands called Carpal Tunnel Syndrome. All of these changes, which result from working at a desk job, can be improved dramatically by doing - you guessed it - exercises and stretches.

The first muscle of concern is the biceps. The biceps runs from the top of the humerus and the coracoid process of the shoulder blade, down the front of the upper arm and across the elbow joint to attach to the radius bone of the forearm. When the biceps muscle contracts, it causes the elbow to bend. Working at a desk most of the day with your elbow bent 90° results in a chronically tight biceps muscle. When your biceps is tight, it can cause discomfort in your arm and can interfere with normal shoulder movement.

The next muscle is the triceps muscle. The triceps is the large muscle group that runs down the back of your arm to attach to the ulna bone at the elbow. Like the biceps, the triceps muscle attaches to both the humerus bone as well as the shoulder blade, making both of these muscles important for proper shoulder function. Because of the type of work involved at a desk job, the triceps muscle rarely gets used, so it becomes weak. This weakness, in conjunction with the tightness of the biceps, can lead to shoulder problems as well as pain and chronic tightness in the arms.

The forearm extensors are a group of muscles that run down the back of the forearm and attach to the back of the hand and fingers. These muscles are responsible for straightening the fingers and bending the hand back at the wrist. On the front of the forearm are the flexor muscles. These muscles are responsible for allowing you to close your hand and bend your hand forward at the wrist. People who do a lot of work with their hands, especially typing and writing, tend to have a lot of tightness in these muscles. This chronic tightness can contribute to a condition called Carpal Tunnel Syndrome, where the nerves that feed the hand become irritated and painful.

Ergonomically-correct workspace design can go a long way toward reducing the degree of muscle tightness and pain in your arms, wrists and hands, but when the Desk Distortion Posture is the cause of the problem, the only way to correct it is by doing your daily exercises and stretches.

Anatomy of the Arms

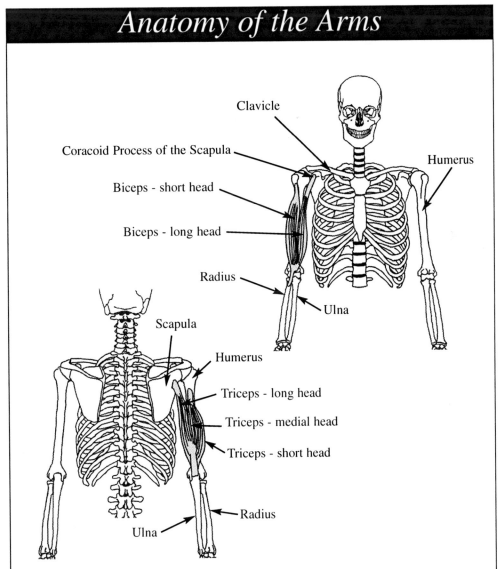

Clavicle

Coracoid Process of the Scapula

Humerus

Biceps - short head

Biceps - long head

Radius

Ulna

Scapula

Humerus

Triceps - long head

Triceps - medial head

Triceps - short head

Radius

Ulna

The two primary muscles of the upper arm are the biceps and the triceps. Because those who work at a desk job usually hold their arms in front of them with their elbows bent, the biceps muscle becomes shortened and chronically tight. This tightness contributes to pain in the shoulder as well as in the forearms and even in the hands. In addition, the chronic tightness in the biceps leads to weakness in the triceps due to reciprocal inhibition, which we talked about in Chapter 1.

Dumbbell Curls

Benefits:	Biceps Strength
Equipment Needed:	Pair of Dumbbells
Time / Repetitions:	10 - 15 Repetitions for Each Arm

The Dumbbell Curl is the simplest, most effective way to improve the strength in the biceps muscle. To do this exercise, start by standing up straight and holding one dumbbell in each hand; palms facing forward. Using only the muscles in your arm, lift the weight up to your shoulder by bending your elbow. Once you raise the weight as far as you can, gently lower it back down again. One entire repetition should take 3 - 4 seconds.

It is important when doing this exercise to keep your elbows locked to your side and not move them forward or backward - that's cheating. The other important thing is to keep your body from swaying back when you raise the dumbbell - that's also cheating. My favorite way to do this exercise is to alternate hands so that while I am raising a dumbbell with one hand, I am lowering the dumbbell in the other. But you may prefer to only exercise one arm at a time. Either way is okay as long as you do 10 - 15 repetitions with each arm. As with the other exercises, if you are able to do 16 repetitions, you need to increase the weight you are lifting. If you are unable to do ten repetitions, you will need to decrease the weight you are using.

This exercise is particularly effective in reducing the tightness in your biceps if you immediately follow it up with the Biceps Door Stretch.

Dumbbell Curls

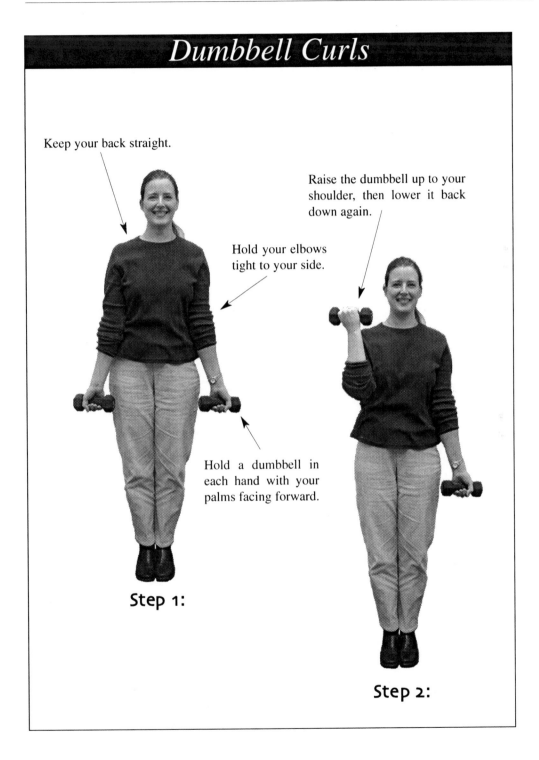

Keep your back straight.

Raise the dumbbell up to your shoulder, then lower it back down again.

Hold your elbows tight to your side.

Hold a dumbbell in each hand with your palms facing forward.

Step 1:

Step 2:

Chair Dips

Benefits:	Triceps Strength
Equipment Needed:	Chair
Time / Repetitions:	10 - 15 Repetitions

This exercise does wonders for the strength of the triceps muscle and, to a lesser degree, the muscles in the front of the shoulder. To do this exercise, start by leaning against the edge of your chair, place your hands on either side and grip the arms of your chair. Move your hips about 12" - 18" away from the edge of the chair by moving your feet forward, while keeping your arms straight and your hands gripping the arms of the chair. Keeping your back straight and your head up, lower your hips as far as you can toward the floor by bending your elbows, then straighten your arms to lift yourself up again. Repeat this exercise for a total of 10 - 15 repetitions.

Depending on your condition, you may find this exercise to be very difficult. Don't worry if you cannot do ten repetitions, or even five repetitions for that matter, when you first try this exercise. If you just keep doing Chair Dips, you will gradually become stronger and they will become easier.

One trick that works well when you cannot do ten repetitions of a particular exercise is to break up the routine into smaller chunks. You may want to do five repetitions, take a short break, then do five more. You can even break it into two-repetition chunks if you have to, and do two repetitions five times throughout the day.

Chair Dips

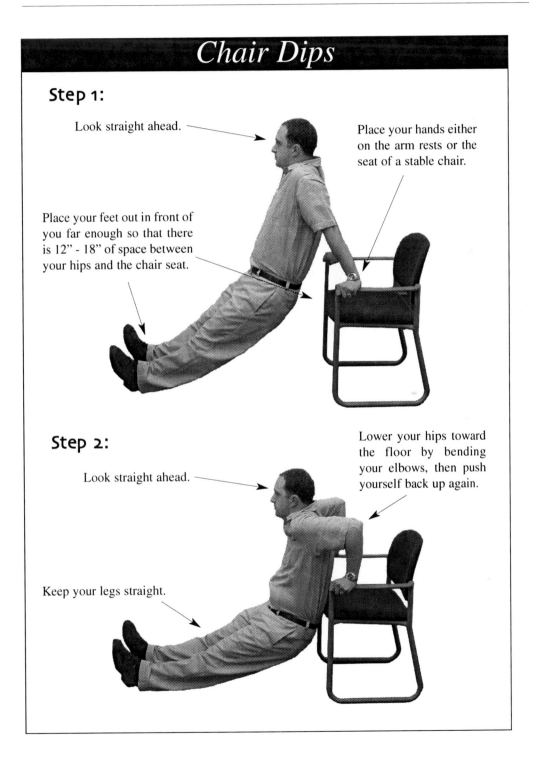

Step 1:

Look straight ahead.

Place your hands either on the arm rests or the seat of a stable chair.

Place your feet out in front of you far enough so that there is 12" - 18" of space between your hips and the chair seat.

Step 2:

Look straight ahead.

Lower your hips toward the floor by bending your elbows, then push yourself back up again.

Keep your legs straight.

The Overhead Press

Benefits: Shoulder and Triceps Strength

Equipment Needed: Pair of Dumbbells

Time / Repetitions: 10 - 15 Repetitions

The Overhead Press is a great overall exercise to improve the strength in the triceps and shoulders. Begin by grasping a pair of dumbbells and raising them up to your shoulders, palms facing forward as shown in the picture on the opposite page. Raise the weights above your head by straightening your arms and bring the weights together so that they touch. Then gently lower the weights back down to the level of your shoulders. Repeat for a total of 10 - 15 repetitions.

If you have never done this exercise before, your arms may feel fairly wobbly and uncoordinated. This is normal and will go away after a couple of weeks of doing the exercise. It is also common for people who have not done this exercise before to feel like their muscles are not getting a very good workout. This happens because you are asking your muscles to work in a way that they are not used to, so they will be a bit uncoordinated. Just keep doing the exercise and you will eventually feel your muscles begin to get a good workout.

It is important when doing the Overhead Press that two basic safety rules are followed. The first is that you should not use a weight that is too heavy for you. If you cannot do ten repetitions, you need to use a lighter weight. The second is that you should not use dumbbells that have removable plates. Instead, use solid-cast, one-piece dumbbells that cannot come apart and cause injury when they are raised above your head.

The Overhead Press

Raise the dumbbells above your head as high as you can until they gently touch.

Hold a dumbbell in each hand with your palms facing forward.

Sit up straight.

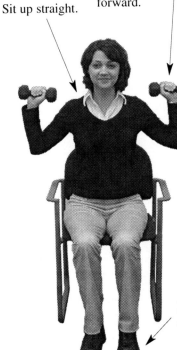

Place your feet flat on the floor.

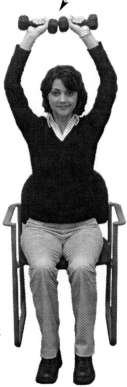

Step 1:

Step 2:

The Biceps Door Stretch

Benefits: Biceps Flexibility

Equipment Needed: Doorway

Time / Repetitions: 30 - 45 Seconds on Each Side

The Biceps Door Stretch is a very effective way to decrease the tightness in the biceps muscles. To do this stretch, begin by gripping the frame of a door so that your thumb points toward the floor as shown in the picture on the opposite page. Slide your hand up to just below the level of your shoulder. Turn your body so that your arm is directly behind you and your shoulders are parallel to the wall. Gently push your pelvis forward until you feel a stretch in your upper arm. Hold the stretch for 30 - 45 seconds, then switch arms and do the same. When you switch arms, you will have to move to the other side of the door frame.

This stretch can be a bit tricky. If you do not feel a stretch in your arm, you are probably doing one of two things incorrectly. The first and most common mistake that most people make is that their shoulders are not parallel to the wall where the door is located. Make sure that your shoulders are lined up with the wall and not in a straight line with your arm. The second mistake is not raising your hand high enough behind you. This is easily corrected by simply sliding your hand up further. As long as your shoulders are square with the wall, you will eventually reach a point where you feel a stretch in your biceps muscle.

You can make this stretch even more effective by performing it immediately following your Dumbbell Curls when your muscles are nice and warm.

The Biceps Door Stretch

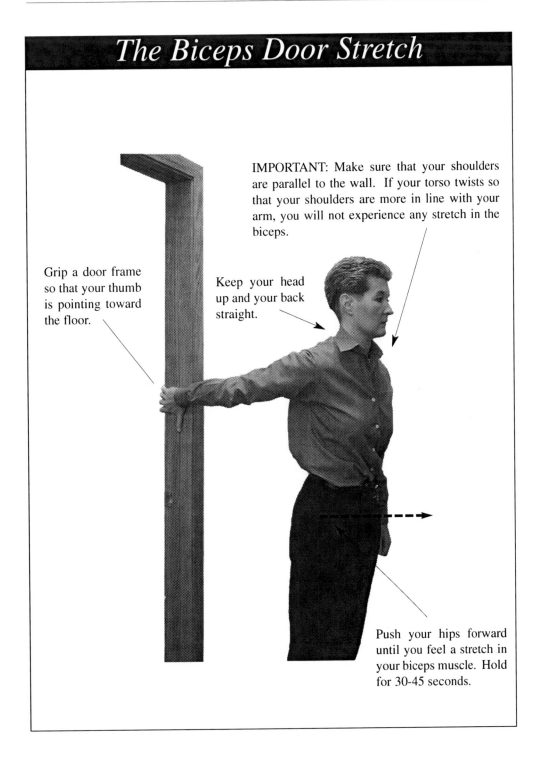

IMPORTANT: Make sure that your shoulders are parallel to the wall. If your torso twists so that your shoulders are more in line with your arm, you will not experience any stretch in the biceps.

Grip a door frame so that your thumb is pointing toward the floor.

Keep your head up and your back straight.

Push your hips forward until you feel a stretch in your biceps muscle. Hold for 30-45 seconds.

The Wrist Stretch

Benefits:	Wrist and Forearm Flexibility
Equipment Needed:	None
Time / Repetitions:	30 - 45 Seconds

The Wrist Stretch is designed to decrease the tension in your forearms and wrists. To do this stretch straighten out one of your arms and allow your wrist to relax. Take your other hand and gently pull your wrist into further flexion as shown in Step 1 in the picture on the opposite page. Hold this stretch for 30 - 45 seconds, then switch directions and pull your hand upwards to stretch the forearm flexors. Hold this stretch for 30 - 45 seconds, then switch hands.

To get the most out of this stretch, it is best to do it at least twice per day; three times would be even better. Be careful not to pull too hard on your hand and over stretch the muscles in your forearms. Those muscles are fairly small and can be strained easily.

If you suffer from Carpal Tunnel Syndrome, this stretch may cause some tingling in your hands. Minor tingling is probably not a major concern and should improve by doing this stretch after a few days. However, if the pain or tingling in your hands is moderate to severe, only do the Wrist Stretch to the point where the pain begins, then back off a bit.

When you experience tingling in your hands by doing the Wrist Stretch, it indicates that the median nerve which runs through the center of your wrist, is being pinched. You don't want to pinch it too much or you may cause the nerve to become irritated or injured. So remember a little tingling is okay when doing the Wrist Stretch, but a lot of tingling or pain is a sign that you are overdoing it a bit.

The Wrist Stretch

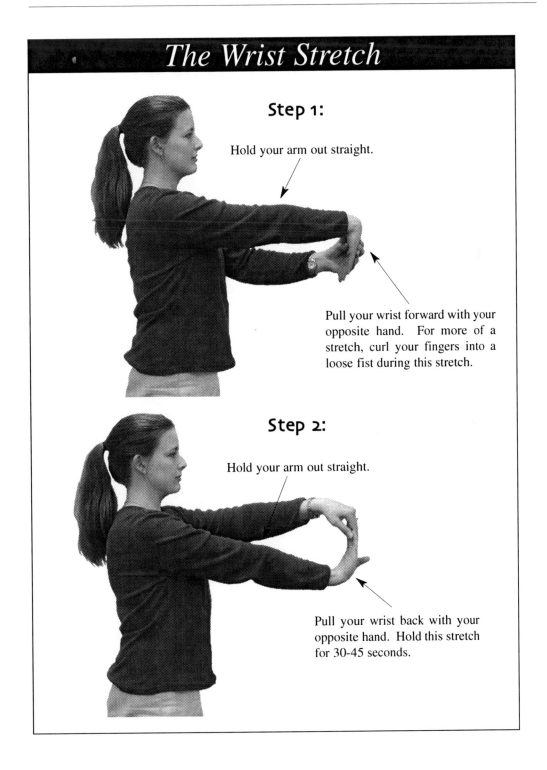

Step 1:

Hold your arm out straight.

Pull your wrist forward with your opposite hand. For more of a stretch, curl your fingers into a loose fist during this stretch.

Step 2:

Hold your arm out straight.

Pull your wrist back with your opposite hand. Hold this stretch for 30-45 seconds.

The Prayer Stretch

Benefits: Hand and Wrist Flexibility

Equipment Needed: None

Time / Repetitions: 30 - 45 Seconds, then 20 - 30 Seconds

This stretch is great for decreasing the tension in your hands, fingers and wrists. To do the Prayer Stretch, start by spreading your fingers apart a little and touching the fingertips of your two hands together, keeping your fingers straight. Gently push your palms toward each other while lowering your hands just enough to keep your palms from touching, as shown in the picture on the opposite page. At this point, you should feel a stretch in your hands and wrists. Holding the separation between your palms, rotate your wrists so that at one extreme your thumb is level with your stomach and at the other extreme your little finger touches your beltline; as shown in the pictures on the opposite page.

This stretch really needs to be done gently and often. The muscles and connective tissues in your hands, fingers and wrists are very small and prone to strain, so go for a good stretch, but don't overdo it. Since people with desk jobs tend to hold their hands in a semi-closed position most of the day, this stretch will really help re-establish normal flexibility.

The Prayer Stretch

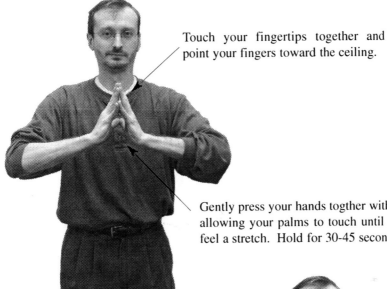

Touch your fingertips together and point your fingers toward the ceiling.

Gently press your hands togther without allowing your palms to touch until you feel a stretch. Hold for 30-45 seconds.

Step 1:

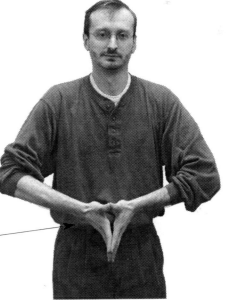

Keeping the pressure on your fingertips, rotate your wrists so that your fingers point toward the floor. Hold for an additional 20-30 seconds.

Step 2:

Deskercise Aerobics

So far we have discussed exercises and stretches to improve strength and flexibility. In this section we will discuss activities which will help to improve your coordination, circulation, metabolism and overall cardiovascular health - aerobics. Aerobic exercises are simply low-intensity, long-duration exercises that primarily use the larger muscles of the body to improve overall body conditioning. Examples of aerobic exercises are bicycling, running, swimming, cross-country skiing and dancing. What all of these exercises have in common is that they are full-body exercises that are done at a low intensity for an extended period, say 15 - 60 minutes, rather than just 10 - 15 repetitions.

By incorporating at least 15 minutes of aerobic exercise into your daily routine, you will experience a host of benefits, such as increased concentration, decreased pain, weight loss and an overall improved feeling of well-being. Doing this minimal amount of aerobic exercise should not be difficult as long as you can walk. If your place of employment has a flight of stairs that you can climb, even better. The two exercises that we will describe in this section are stair-climbing and power walking.

Power Walking

Benefits:	Aerobic Training
Equipment Needed:	None
Time / Repetitions:	15 Minutes

Power Walking is much like regular walking, only faster. Contrary to what most people believe, leisure walking is not the best exercise. As a matter of fact, walking at a normal pace has very little exercise value for people who have relatively good health. In order for walking to have maximum value as an exercise, it has to be done at a pace that is faster than normal. You can increase the exercise value even more by carrying light dumbbells in your hands while you Power Walk.

The benefits of Power Walking include cardiovascular conditioning, such as normalized blood pressure, better circulation and decreased serum cholesterol, increased metabolism to help maintain a healthy body weight, and improved mental functioning, including better concentration, improved mood, decreased stress and more restful sleep. In order to experience these benefits, it is important to do some form of aerobic exercise, such as Power Walking, every day; or at least five days per week.

Stair Climbers

Benefits:	Aerobic Training and Leg Strength
Equipment Needed:	Flight of Stairs
Time / Repetitions:	15 Minutes

Stair Climbers have all of the same benefits as Power Walking, but with the additional benefit of improving leg and hip strength. They are much more intense than Power Walking so they may not be the best exercise with which to begin, unless you have previously exercised regularly. A better approach for a beginner is to Power Walk five days per week for one month, then slowly start to integrate some Stair Climbers with your walk. For example, you may start by climbing for one minute up and down a flight of stairs for one week, as part of your walking routine; then increase the time for Stair Climbers to two minutes, then to three, then four minutes, etc.

If you have knee problems, Stair Climbers may be a problem for you. It is surprising to most people to learn that climbing up a flight of stairs is easier on your knees than walking down the steps. This is because when you are walking up a flight of stairs, the big muscles of the quadriceps contract to stabilize your knees. But when you walk down stairs, the only thing stabilizing the knee is a small ligament that lies deep within your knee joint called the cruciate ligament. For this reason, you can be more aggressive while climbing stairs as long as you are more controlled and gentle while walking back down again. If your knees tend to pop and crackle while you do Stair Climbers, you may consider taking glucosamine sulfate, a nutritional supplement that can help to strengthen your cartilage.

6 Changing Unhealthy Lifestyle Habits

So far we have covered a lot of material about exercises and stretches to keep your body strong, flexible and pain-free. But there is more to being healthy than just exercising and stretching. Regular chiropractic care, eating a healthy diet, taking vitamin supplements, keeping your weight under control and stress management are all part of an overall wellness lifestyle that, if followed, results in a longer, healthier and pain-free life. Unfortunately, few people have developed these healthy lifestyle habits. Consequently, they are at an increased risk of heart disease, cancer, depression, chronic pain, obesity and a whole host of other preventable conditions.

In this chapter we will talk about healthy lifestyle habits and how to break free from unhealthy habits. Let's start with the importance of routine chiropractic care.

Chiropractic Care

Routine chiropractic care is one of the simplest ways to maintain the health of your body. Numerous research studies have shown that people who

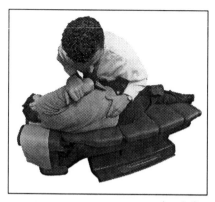

receive regular chiropractic care suffer fewer illnesses, injuries and degenerative diseases, and they report a better overall quality of life. In spite of the health benefits of chiropractic care, many people have never been to a chiropractor, most often because they don't really understand what chiropractic care is all about. Two of the most common reasons cited for why people don't seek chiropractic care are either because they have heard somewhere that it is dangerous or that onece you start going to a chiropractor, you have to continue going forever.

"Once you start going to a chiropractor, you have to keep going to them forever" is a statement that I frequently hear when the topic of chiropractic care comes up in conversation. This statement is only partly true. You only have to continue going to the chiropractor as long as you wish to maintain the health of your neuromusculoskeletal system. Going to a chiropractor is much like going to the dentist, exercising at a gym or eating a healthier diet. If you routinely go to the dentist throughout your whole life, your teeth will likely stay strong and healthy. But if you only go to the dentist when your teeth hurt, the long-term health of your teeth will suffer.

If you go to the gym and begin working out, you will only maintain the benefits of exercise as long as you make it part of your routine. If you exercise for a while and get your body into shape, only to stop exercising again, you will lose most of the health benefits you gained. If you go on a healthy diet and stop consuming junk food, you will soon feel better, look better and have more energy; that is, as long as you make the diet part of your routine.

The same is true with chiropractic care. Although you can enjoy the benefits of chiropractic care even if you are only treated for a short time, the real benefits come into play when you make chiropractic care a part of your lifestyle.

One other statement that I frequently hear is that chiropractic care is dangerous, especially neck adjustments. While it would be untrue to say that chiropractic adjustments have no risk, it is also untrue to say that they are dangerous. As a matter of fact, you are over a thousand times more likely to suffer a negative reaction to taking an aspirin than you are to suffer a negative reaction to a chiropractic adjustment.

The bottom line is that chiropractic care is a safe, effective treatment for a wide range of physical complaints, such as headaches, neck pain, low back pain, Carpal Tunnel Syndrome, Thoracic Outlet Syndrome, stomach and gastrointestinal complaints, wrist, elbow and shoulder pain, knee, hip and ankle pain, scoliosis, otitis media, and a host of other problems. While most of these disorders resolve within a few weeks or months, routine chiropractic care will help ensure optimal health for life.

Eating Fruits and Vegetables

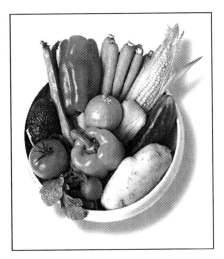

People know that they should eat more fruit and vegetables in their diet, but most don't. It seems lately that the four major food groups of the American diet have gone from dairy, fruits and vegetables, grains and meat to sugar, fat, salt and caffeine. Because of the easy availability of fast foods and snack foods, we have lost our taste for fruits and vegetables; especially vegetables. It is not uncommon for many people to go for weeks on end without consuming a single serving of fresh vegetables. This is not good.

The human body evolved with a diet high in fruits and vegetables, and is dependent on many of the compounds unique to plant foods in order to operate correctly. If you don't consume enough of these plant compounds, your energy level will suffer along with your overall health. Most people are shocked at how much better they feel when they cut down on the fast foods and snack foods and increase their fruit and vegetable intake.

If you find it difficult to work in several servings of fruits and vegetables into your routine every day, you may find it helpful to supplement your diet with what is called a "greens" supplement; which is a highly concentrated powder of fruits, vegetables and antioxidants. On my website, www.drtodd.com, I list the information about one product which is of unusually good quality and is the one I recommend to my patients, called Super Fruits and Greens.

Increasing your consumption of fruits and vegetables is an important way to improve your overall health. The key is to make it part of your lifestyle - to make it a new habit.

Vitamin Supplements

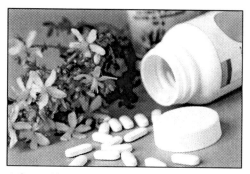

During one of my graduate nutrition courses, my professor posed a challenge to the class: Construct a 2000 calorie-per-day diet that at least met the Recommended Dietary Allowances (RDA), for vitamins and minerals without the use of supplements. After all, we have always heard that if you eat a well-balanced diet, you don't need to take vitamin supplements right? My professor was putting that statement to the test.

To everyone's surprise, none of us was able to come up with a sustainable daily diet that met the minimum requirements for vitamin and mineral intake. The problem was not with getting the minimum vitamin intake; that was relatively easy. The challenge was getting enough of a few very important minerals, especially zinc. Unless you eat oysters or dark turkey meat every day, it is impossible to get the minimum RDA of zinc through diet alone.

So, it is not possible to get everything that you need from diet alone. But how could this be? Certainly people have lived on this planet for a long time and must have been able to get everything they needed from diet alone. The answer has to do with modern farming techniques, fertilizers and environmental stresses.

Following the Second World War, chemical manufacturers were sitting on huge stockpiles of phosphates and nitrates that were initially intended for use in explosives. They discovered that when they spread these same phosphates and nitrates on the soil where plants were growing, the plants grew bigger and looked healthier. Thus began the boom of the fertilizer industry.

The problem with modern fertilizers is that they don't replace soil trace minerals, such as chromium, zinc and copper, as does cow manure and other natural fertilizers. Over time, these trace minerals become more and more depleted from the soil and, consequently, our food supply becomes more depleted as well. The bottom line is that in order to get enough trace minerals in our diet to at least meet the minimum RDAs, it is necessary to take a good quality supplement.

Another argument for taking multivitamin and mineral supplements is that there is substantial evidence that taking doses of a class of nutrients called antioxidants that far exceed the RDA minimums can help prevent heart disease, help to mitigate some of the detrimental effects of diabetes and help to promote healthy immune function.

Smoking Cessation

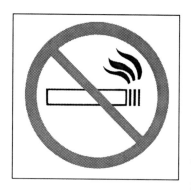

If you smoke, you should stop. It's not good for you. Smoking throughout the day is akin to living inside a burning building. Smoking degrades the collagen of your skin, causing premature wrinkling, destroys the cells inside your lungs, promotes heart disease, cataracts and cancer because of the oxidizing radicals released into the blood stream and can contribute to back pain by dehydrating the spinal discs.

People stop smoking every day and so can you. Some people find acupuncture to be very helpful at reducing cravings and many people have used nicotine patches for the same reason. But these are not as important as your unswerving, absolute commitment to do whatever it takes to not smoke today. Just limit your not smoking to today only. You can tell yourself that you can have a cigarette tomorrow if you just make it through today. Tomorrow morning when you wake up, tell yourself the same thing. I have known many addicts who have successfully kicked their alcohol, heroine or cocaine addictions this way. Kicking any addiction is tough. You must expect to feel stressed, anxious and irritable at first. To expect anything else is unreasonable. But you can also expect that over time it will become easier and easier to not smoke.

The Battle of the Bulge

The sad fact is that more Americans are overweight than ever before. Being overweight not only affects how you look, but it affects your mental state, how well you sleep, your blood pressure, circulating blood sugar levels and even your mental and emotional health.

There are two different components that are important to understand if you are one of those people who would like to lose weight. These are metabolism and diet. Let's start by talking about metabolism.

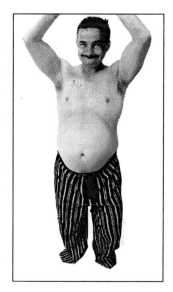

Most people are familiar with the word metabolism and understand that it has something to do with the way that the body processes food. People with a high metabolism burn up more of the food they eat and tend to be thinner than those who have a low or slow metabolism. The key is to raise your metabolism in order to burn more of the calories your body takes in so you can be thinner. The most powerful metabolism booster available is exercise.

When you exercise, the body responds by building new muscle tissue, increasing the blood supply to the muscles and strengthening your bones. All of this takes energy, and a lot of it. Professional bodybuilders can consume in excess of 10,000 calories in a single day - about as much as some people eat in a week - and not get fat because they exercise so intensely. If you want to lose weight, elevating your metabolism is key, and the most effective way to elevate your metabolism is to exercise.

Unfortunately, not all activities are intense enough to elevate your metabolism. You must exercise at an intensity level that leaves you a bit out of breath. This may include going on a 15 minute Power Walk or pushing yourself a little bit extra when doing your Deskercises. A leisurely walk through a shopping mall will not be intense enough.

Diet is the other part of the equation for weight loss. If you want to lose weight, it is important to control what you are eating. If you eat a lot of food every day and your activity level is not high enough to burn all those calories,

1e extra calories you consume will be stored as fat. This means that you will probably have to reduce the total number of calories you consume every day by reducing the amount of food you eat. But if you reduce your food intake too much, it can also cause problems.

One problem that occurs when you reduce your food intake too much is that your metabolism slows down, which is something you want to avoid. When you restrict calories to lose weight, you not only lose fat, but you also lose muscle. This muscle loss results in a slower metabolism. Once you come off your diet and resume your normal eating pattern, you will not only gain all of the body fat back that you had before, but since your metabolism is even slower due to muscle loss, you will most likely end up heavier than when you started. This is what leads to the yo-yo effect in trying to lose weight through dieting.

The key to dieting for weight loss is to simply avoid certain foods such as fast food of any kind and avoid soft drinks, fruit juices, candy and sweets of any kind. Four to six times per day, you should eat one serving of protein - cottage cheese, meat, fish or eggs - and one serving of complex carbohydrate - vegetables, rice, corn, legumes or fruit.

One serving is roughly equivalent to the size of the palm of your hand. So each meal should have approximately a palm-sized serving of protein and a palm-sized serving of complex carbohydrate. If you follow this way of eating six days a week, allowing one day per week as a day where you can eat as much of whatever you want, you will avoid the potential negative effects of too much calorie restriction while still controlling your food intake to a healthy level.

If you combine this style of eating with daily exercise, you will begin to develop a healthy and trim physique and decrease your risk of numerous illnesses, such as Type II diabetes, heart disease, and cancer.

Heart Health Facts

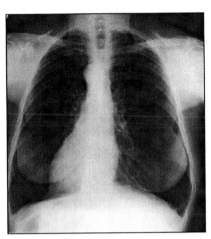

Heart disease is currently the number-one killer of adults in the United States. This is unfortunate because most heart disease is caused by poor lifestyle choices. The four big lifestyle changes you can make to ensure to maximize the health of your heart are exercise, maintaining a healthy body weight, taking a high quality vitamin supplement and stopping smoking.

Just as exercise is important to the health of your neuromusculoskeletal system, it is also critical to the health of your heart. When you regularly exercise, your body becomes much more efficient at using oxygen and burning calories and your blood pressure is normalized. This decreases the stress on your heart.

Another easy way to reduce the stress on your heart is to decrease the amount of body fat you carry around. It takes approximately one mile of additional blood vessels to supply one pound of additional fat. If you are twenty, thirty or fifty pounds overweight, it is easy to see how that extra body fat can place an undue burden on your heart.

Vitamins E, C and folic acid are the three most important nutritional supplements to take for your heart. Vitamin E is a powerful fat-soluble antioxidant which helps to prevent the cholesterol in your blood from becoming oxidized. High cholesterol levels in the blood, *per se*, are not that big of a deal. Cholesterol only becomes dangerous when it interacts with an oxidizing radical. Vitamin E helps to prevent this.

Vitamin C is important to help strengthen the walls of the arteries and prevent the development of cholesterol plaques inside the coronary arteries. Did you know that the arteries that are the most likely to develop cholesterol deposits are the ones that are close to the heart? The reason is that when the heart contracts, it pushes blood out with a great degree of force. If the walls of the arteries which are closest to the heart are not as strong as they should be, they will tend to momentarily stretch out like a balloon and cause small tears to the inside arterial wall as the rush of blood from the heart passes by. These small tears serve as a place where platelets and cholesterol form deposits. High levels of vitamin C reduce the tears in the arteries by strengthening the collagen tissues around the arteries, keeping them from expanding too much as blood pulses through.

The third vitamin which is important is one of the B-vitamins called folic acid. Folic acid, also called folacin, is important for reducing the level of homocysteine in the blood. Homocysteine is a metabolic by-product which can contribute significantly to the development of heart disease.

So, when you take your multivitamin while you are on your way to do your exercises, make sure that it contains at least 400 IU of vitamin E, at least 500 mg of vitamin C (1000 is even better) and 40 mcg of folic acid.

Reducing Stress

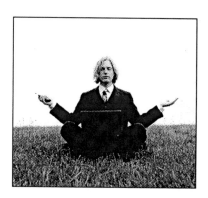

In the past couple of decades there has been a lot of fascinating research into the connection between the mind and the body. It turns out that your emotions and your mood have a tremendous impact on your physical state. People who are stressed suffer from disturbed sleep and supressed immune function, as well as an increased risk of heart disease, depression, high blood pressure and cognitive impairment.

By getting physically active, you can decrease your levels of anxiety and stress and elevate your moods. Numerous studies have shown that people who begin exercise programs, either at home or at work, demonstrate a marked improvement in their ability to concentrate, are able to sleep better, suffer from fewer illnesses, suffer from less pain and report a much higher quality of life than those who do not exercise. This is even true of people who had not begun an exercise program until they were in their 40s, 50s, 60s or even 70s. So if you want to feel better and improve your quality of life, get active!

Avoiding Sugar

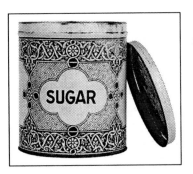

In a recent study done by the USDA, it was reported that the average American consumes 134 pounds of refined sugar every year, or approximately 20 teaspoons of sugar per day. As hard as this may be to believe, consider the following facts:

- A 12 oz. can of Pepsi contains 10 teaspoons of sugar
- A 2 oz. package of candy contains 11 teaspoons of sugar
- A 16 oz. cup of lemonade contains 13 teaspoons of sugar
- A cup of Frosted Flakes cereal contains 4 teaspoons of sugar

This high level of sugar intake is very unhealthy and contributes to obesity, Type II diabetes, heart disease due to elevated triglycerides, kidney stones, dental caries, chronic tiredness and reactive hypoglycemia. Decreasing your sugar intake is as simple as avoiding foods which are high in refined sugars, such as soft drinks, candy, cake, donuts as well as most condiments.

When you purchase purchase sweetened food, look for products that are sweetened with apple juice or stevia, rather than sugar or high-fructose corn syrup.

Drinking Clean Water

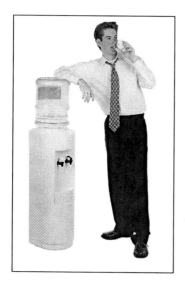

Drinking an adequate amount of clean water every day is one of the most overlooked, but simplest ways of keeping your body healthy. Water is used to help the body cleanse itself from toxins and metabolic waste. Although drinking water has become more popular over the past several years, many people still do not consume enough water. Instead, they drink coffee, tea, juices and soft drinks and figure that they get enough fluids. It is true that when you drink these things you are consuming water. However, along with the water, you are also consuming a lot of other stuff that the body will need to ultimately eliminate, so the potential beneficial effect of the water is negated. To make matters worse, drinks that contain caffeine, such as coffee, tea and soft drinks, actually cause more water loss than the amount of water they contain, resulting in a net loss of water.

Ideally, the average person should consume around ten cups of water per day, or just over a half gallon. Some of this water is found in the food and beverages you consume, so you don't have to drink an entire half-gallon of water every day. What I tell my patients to do is to buy a 1.5 liter bottle of water from the local grocery store and to drink that amount of water every day. If you exercise heavily, you may have to drink two of those 1.5 liter bottles of water each day. By drinking enough water, you will be helping your body to remain healthy. It is by far the cheapest health insurance you can buy.

The Hazards of Television

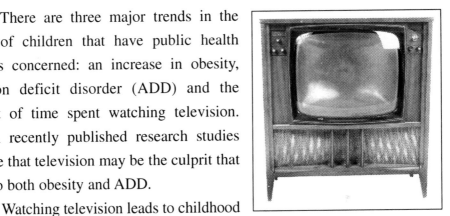

There are three major trends in the health of children that have public health workers concerned: an increase in obesity, attention deficit disorder (ADD) and the amount of time spent watching television. Several recently published research studies indicate that television may be the culprit that leads to both obesity and ADD.

Watching television leads to childhood obesity in two ways. First, for every hour that a kid is sitting in front of the television, they are not outside running around, climbing trees and playing with their friends. This results in that child burning fewer calories through exercise as well as a reduction in his or her overall metabolism. Also, a number of studies have shown that children who watch television just eat more food.

Watching television also has detrimental effects on the cognitive functioning in kids. Studies have shown that children who watch more than two hours of television per day struggle more with aggressive behavioral problems, difficulty in concentrating, sleep disturbances and a dramatic increased risk of alcohol consumption as teenagers. Although most studies have been conducted on children, other studies have shown that the results are just as valid for adolescents and adults as well. These negative effects can be explained by understanding the effect television has on the brain.

Broadcast television in the United States has a particular frequency of flicker that cannot be seen, but has an effect on brain function. A number of studies measured brain wave activity in people while they watch television. During these studies it was noticed that the brain waves in people watching television were similar to people who were in a trance. This trance-like state is associated with a decrease in the function of the cerebral cortex; the critical thinking part of the brain. When people are in this trance-like state for several hours per day, it becomes more difficult to focus their attention and control their impulses.

The American Academy of Pediatrics recommends that children watch no more than two hours of television per day, although it would be better to reduce this even further. Many health experts are now encouraging parents to completely eliminate watching television for children under the age of seven, until their brains have the chance to develop a bit more.

How to Change Unhealthy Habits

There are three things that have to happen to successfully change a habit. The first is to make a decision to change. When you make a decision, you are committing that you are willing to go to any lengths to make your wishes come true. This means that you will need to completely eliminate the word 'try' from your vocabulary. When you say "I'll try to do my exercises," you are leaving an open door to not doing them. Then in your mind, if you don't do your exercises, that's

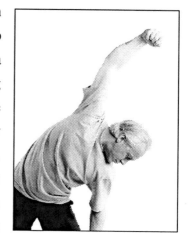

okay becuase you only said you would "try" to do them. If you want to successfully change your habits to live a healthier life, you cannot leave an open door to your old habits. You need to just do it, just make a decision and not look back.

The second thing is to act "as if." Whenever you change what you are doing, it will feel unnatural. It may feel like you are doing something wrong, funny, or something that is just not you. In a way you are right. When you change a habit, you are by definition acting in a way that is 'just not you.' But in a very short time, it will feel normal and it will seem strange that you ever acted any different. Changing habits is like starting a new job, the first couple of weeks are stressful and disorienting, but if you just hang in there, you will feel at home before you know it.

The third and hardest thing that is important to do when you change your bad habits is to not believe everything that you think. The mind is a very powerful justifier. It tells you over and over again why you are justified in thinking and acting in a certain way. If you decide to quit eating so much sugar, it will take a while before your mind gets used to that idea. In the mean time, you may experience thoughts like "oh, don't make such a big deal out of not eating so much sugar, everybody else eats it," or "who are you kidding, you have always eaten a lot of sugar, that's just who you are." When you hear messages like this bubbling up into your consciousness, just remember that you cannot believe everything you think. As your habits change and you become healthier, your thinking will change right along with it.

For More Information

For more information on these and other health topics, please visit my website at:

www.drtodd.com

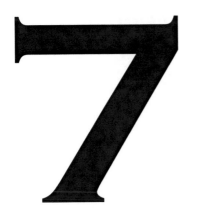

7 Doing The Deskercise Program

Recall from earlier that people who work at desk jobs tend to have a particular collection of physical changes called the Desk Distortion Posture. This pattern includes weakened rhomboid muscles in the mid-back, shoulders and head carried forward, weakened abdominal muscles, chronically tight trapezius and levator scapulae muscles in the upper back as well as chronically tight psoas muscles in the low back. In order to be effective, your exercise program should be based on a series of exercises to specifically target these problems.

If you look at the chart on the next page, you will notice that there are six exercises that are listed at the top for you to do each day. These "Deskercise Six," as I call them, directly counteract the effects of working at a desk job. Below the Deskercise Six are several spaces for you to add additional exercises based on your own needs and goals. I suggest that you try a number of different exercises and see which ones you like and add those to your daily routine. I also included a workout chart that does not contain the top six exercises in case you are one of those who are unable to do one or more of those exercises. If this is the case you can design your own program from scratch. Photocopy

The Basic Deskercise Program

Monday	Tuesday	Wednesday	Thursday	Friday
Dumbbell Row	Dumbbell Row	Dumbbell Row	Dumbbell Row	Dumbbell Row
Stick-Em Up Stretch	Stick-Em Up Stretch	Stick-Em Up Stretch	Stick-Em Up Stretch	Stick-Em Up Stretch
Pelvic Tilts	Pelvic Tilts	Pelvic Tilts	Pelvic Tilts	Pelvic Tilts
Psoas Stretch	Psoas Stretch	Psoas Stretch	Psoas Stretch	Psoas Stretch
Wall Posture Exercise	Wall Posture Exercise	Wall Posture Exercise	Wall Posture Exercise	Wall Posture Exercise
Power Walking	Power Walking	Power Walking	Power Walking	Power Walking
Personal Deskercises	Personal Deskercises	Personal Deskercises	Personal Deskercises	Personal Deskercises

whichever chart you are going to use and put it up in a conspicuous place on your wall so that you see it every day.

It is a good idea to keep a daily record of what exercises you do, what food you eat as well as any other information that pertains to your health, such as tobacco and alcohol use. There are a couple of reasons to do this. First, by writing down what you do every day, it keeps you on track. If everything is written down, it's easier to look at what you have done, what has worked for you and what has not.

Another reason to write everything down is that it helps to cement your new Deskercise program into a habit. Experience has shown that it takes about 21 days of following a particular pattern of behavior for that behavior to become a habit. Once it is a habit, it is very easy to continue. Writing down your exercises every day helps to speed the process up a bit. On page 157 there is a form that you can use to keep track of your daily progress. Just make a bunch of photocopies, put them in a three-ring binder and keep them at your desk.

If you are one of the millions of people who suffers from headaches, neck or back pain, you can also track the progress of your pain symptoms by taking the Pain Questionnaire in Appendix 2 once a month and placing the results on the Pain Progress Form on page 158.

If you have any questions about the Deskercise program, want more information, or would like to download the forms from this book, please visit my website at: www.drtodd.com.

GOOD LUCK!

My Deskercise Workout

Monday	Tuesday	Wednesday	Thursday	Friday

My Daily Progress

Today's date: _____

Exercise/ Stretch	Repetitions/ Time
1) _____	_____
2) _____	_____
3) _____	_____
4) _____	_____
5) _____	_____
6) _____	_____
7) _____	_____
8) _____	_____
9) _____	_____
10) _____	_____
11) _____	_____
12) _____	_____
13) _____	_____
14) _____	_____

Diet

Meal 1

_____

_____

_____

Meal 2

_____

_____

_____

Meal 3

_____

_____

_____

Meal 4

_____

_____

Today's Success: _____

_____

_____

Goals for Tomorrow: _____

_____

The Pain Progress Form

General Disability

Test date: _____

Score: _____

Low Back Pain

Test date: _____

Score: _____

Neck Pain

Test date: _____

Score: _____

Headaches

Test date: _____

Score: _____

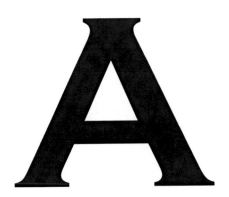 # Appendix 1: The Healthy Lifestyle Questionnaire

The Healthy Lifestyle Questionnaire is a quick and easy way to gauge the overall healthiness of your current lifestyle habits. Next to each statement or question, simply mark the box which most accurately describes you. Once you have finished answering all the questions, you can score your questionnaire by adding up the numbers in the boxes for each of the statements you checked and plotting them on the chart at the end of this section. You can then use this information to look at ways to change some of your unhealthy habits to healthier ones.

General Health

How do you rate your own health?

- ☐ 1 Above average
- ☐ 3 About average
- ☐ 5 Below average

How often do you visit the dentist?

☐1 More than once per year
☐3 About once per year
☐5 Less than once per year

How often do you visit the chiropractor?

☐1 At least once every six weeks
☐3 Only when I need it
☐5 Rarely or never

What is your cholesterol level?

☐1 Below 210
☐3 Above 210
☐5 Never had it checked

How stressful is your day to day life?

☐1 Very low stress
☐3 Occasionally stressful
☐5 Very stressful

Are overweight or underweight?

☐1 No
☐3 Yes, by less than 20 pounds
☐5 Yes, by more than 20 pounds

Nutrition

How often do you take a multivitamin?

☐1 Every day
☐3 Occasionally
☐5 Rarely or never

How often do you consume fast food?

- ☐1 Less than once per week
- ☐3 About once or twice per week
- ☐5 More than twice per week

How many servings of fruits and vegetables do you consume each day?

- ☐1 More than five servings
- ☐3 Three to five servings
- ☐5 Fewer than three servings

How much pure water do you drink each day?

- ☐1 More than 64 oz.
- ☐3 Between 32 oz. and 64 oz.
- ☐5 Less than 32 oz.

How many servings of sweets do you consume each day, such as ice cream, candy, cookies, donuts, etc.?

- ☐1 Less than one
- ☐3 Between one and three
- ☐5 More than three

How often do you eat a high-protein breakfast?

- ☐1 Every day
- ☐3 At least once per week
- ☐5 Rarely or never

Recreation and Activity

Overall, how physically active are you?

- ☐1 Very athletic
- ☐3 Moderately physically active
- ☐5 Mildly physically active

How physically demanding is your job?

- ☐ Moderately demanding
- ☐ Very physically demanding
- ☐ Not very demanding

How many hours per week do you spend doing vigorous exercise?

- ☐ More than four hours
- ☐ Two to four hours
- ☐ Fewer than two hours

How often do you stretch your muscles?

- ☐ Daily
- ☐ Occasionally
- ☐ Rarely or never

How often do you participate in recreational sports, such as golf, swimming, tennis, etc.?

- ☐ At least once a week
- ☐ About once per month
- ☐ Less than once per month

How many miles per week do you run, jog, or briskly walk?

- ☐ More than five miles
- ☐ One to five miles
- ☐ Less than one mile

Other Habits

How often do you use tobacco?

- ☐ Rarely or never
- ☐ Less than once per week
- ☐ At least once per week

How much alcohol do you consume?

1 None or very little

3 Less than one drink per day

5 More than one drink per day

How often do you use recreational drugs, such as marijuana, amphetamines or cocaine?

1 Never

3 Less than once per month

5 At least once per month

How many hours of restful sleep do you get each night?

1 Six to eight hours

3 More than nine hours

5 Five hours or fewer

How is your relationship with the person closest to you?

1 Excellent

3 Occasionally problematic

5 Frequently troubled

How satisfied are you with your life right now?

1 Satisfied

3 Somewhat satisfied

5 Unsatisfied

Do you use stress-relieving medication or alcohol to help you cope with stressful situations?

1 Rarely or never

3 Occasionally

5 Frequently

Turn to the next page to score your questionnaire.

Scoring Your Questionnaire

There is a number inside the square next to each answer you checked. Add up the total for each section and enter them below. Add these numbers together to get your total score.

General Health: _____

Nutrition: _____

Recreation and Activity: _____

Other Habits: _____

Total: _____

Interpreting your score:

101-125 - Poor Lifestyle Habits. You are at a high risk for developing preventible health conditions.

76-100 - Borderline Lifestyle Habits. You have a moderately high risk for developing preventible health conditions.

51-75 - Good Lifestyle Habits. You have a moderately low risk for developing preventible health conditions.

25-50 - Excellent Lifestyle Habits. You have a very low risk of developing preventible health conditions.

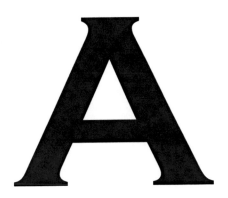

Appendix 2: The Pain Questionnaire

The Pain Questionnaire is a simple tool to help you objectively measure the severity of your pain. By taking this questionnaire on a monthly or bi-monthly basis, it can provide an objective measure of your progress.

To take this questionnaire, simply choose which statement is most true for you in each section. Choosing between statements can sometimes be difficult, especially if you suffer from intermittent pain. If this is the case with you, select the question that most accurately describes the general level of discomfort you have experienced over the previous two weeks.

Once you have finished answering all the questions, you can score your questionnaire by adding up the numbers in the boxes for each of the statements you checked and plotting them on the Pain Progress Form on page 158.

General Disability from Pain

Personal Care

0 The pain comes and goes and is very mild.

1 The pain is constant and is mild in intensity.

2 The pain comes and goes and is moderate in intensity.

3 The pain is constant and is moderate in intensity.

4 The pain comes and goes and is severe.

5 The pain is constant and is severe.

Sleeping

0 The pain is rapidly getting better, or I have no pain when I sleep.

1 The pain fluctuates, but is definitely getting better.

2 The pain is getting better, but very slowly.

3 The pain is neither improving nor worsening.

4 The pain is gradually worsening.

5 The pain is rapidly worsening.

Social Activities

0 My social activities do not cause me any additional pain.

1 My social activities cause me some additional pain.

2 Pain limits my more energetic social activities, such as dancing, exercising, etc.

3 Pain has limited my social activities and I only go out occasionally.

4 Pain restricts my social activities to my home.

5 Pain totally prohibits any kind of social activity.

Housework

0 I am able to perform any housework without pain.

1 I am able to perform any housework, but it causes a mild increase in pain.

2 I am able to perform any housework, but it causes a moderate increase in pain.

3 I am able to do most light and medium housework due to pain.

4 I am only able to do some light housework due to pain.

5 I am unable to perform any housework due to pain.

Work Performance

☐0 I can do as much work as I want without experiencing additional pain.

☐1 I can do my usual work, but pain keeps me from doing more.

☐2 I can only do most of my usual work because of pain.

☐3 I cannot do my usual work.

☐4 Pain keeps me from doing much work at all.

☐5 I am unable to do work of any kind due to pain.

Work Absence

☐0 I never miss work because of pain.

☐1 I never miss work, but am occasionally on light duty due to pain.

☐2 I miss less than one week per year, and often cannot do some of my job.

☐3 I miss more than one week, but less than one month per year due to pain.

☐4 I miss more than one month of work per year due to pain.

☐5 I am disabled due to pain.

Low Back Pain

Pain Intensity

☐0 The pain comes and goes and is very mild.

☐1 The pain is constant and is mild in intensity.

☐2 The pain comes and goes and is moderate in intensity.

☐3 The pain is constant and is moderate in intensity.

☐4 The pain comes and goes and is severe.

☐5 The pain is constant and is severe.

Changing Degree of Pain

☐0 The pain is rapidly getting better, or I have no pain.

☐1 The pain fluctuates, but is definitely getting better.

☐2 The pain is getting better, but very slowly.

☐3 The pain is neither improving nor worsening.

☐4 The pain is gradually worsening.

☐5 The pain is rapidly worsening.

Lifting

0 I can lift heavy weights without additional pain.

1 I can lift heavy weights, but it causes additional pain.

2 I cannot lift heavy weights off the floor due to pain.

3 I cannot lift medium weights off the floor due to pain.

4 I cannot lift anything off the floor, but can lift light weights if they are conveniently positioned.

5 I cannot lift anything, even if it's conveniently positioned, due to pain.

Sitting

0 I can sit in any chair as long as I like without any additional pain.

1 I can only sit in my favorite chair as long as I like without additional pain.

2 Pain prevents me from sitting for more than 1 hour.

3 Pain prevents me from sitting for more than 1/2 hour.

4 Pain prevents me from sitting for more than 15 minutes.

5 I cannot sit at all without increasing my pain immediately.

Standing

0 I can stand as long as I want without pain.

1 Standing causes me some pain, but it does not increase with time.

2 I cannot stand for more than 1 hour without increasing pain.

3 I cannot stand for more than 1/2 hour without increasing pain.

4 I cannot stand for more than 15 minutes without increasing pain.

5 I cannot stand without increasing my pain immediately.

Walking

0 Walking does not cause me any additional pain.

1 Walking causes me some pain, but it does not increase with time.

2 I cannot walk longer than 1 hour without increasing pain.

3 I cannot walk longer than 1/2 hour without increasing pain.

4 I cannot walk longer than 15 minutes without increasing pain.

5 I cannot walk without increasing my pain immediately.

Neck Pain

Pain Intensity
0. The pain comes and goes and is very mild.
1. The pain is constant and is mild in intensity.
2. The pain comes and goes and is moderate in intensity.
3. The pain is constant and is moderate in intensity.
4. The pain comes and goes and is severe.
5. The pain is constant and is severe.

Changing Degree of Pain
0. The pain is rapidly getting better, or I have no pain.
1. The pain fluctuates, but is definitely getting better.
2. The pain is getting better, but very slowly.
3. The pain is neither improving nor worsening.
4. The pain is gradually worsening.
5. The pain is rapidly worsening.

Lifting
0. I can lift heavy weights without additional pain.
1. I can lift heavy weights, but it causes additional pain.
2. I cannot lift heavy weights off the floor due to pain.
3. I cannot lift medium weights off the floor due to pain.
4. I cannot lift anything off the floor, but can lift objects that are waist-high.
5. I cannot lift anything, even if it's conveniently positioned, due to pain.

Reading
0. I can read as much as I want without additional neck pain.
1. I can read as much as I want, but it causes additional neck pain.
2. I can read as much as I want, but I need to take frequent breaks due to pain.
3. I cannot read longer than 1 hour due to neck pain.
4. I cannot read longer than 1/2 hour due to neck pain.
5. I cannot read at all due to neck pain.

Driving

⓪ I can drive as long as I want without any neck pain.

① I can drive as long as I want, but it causes minor additional neck pain.

② I can drive as long as I want, but it causes moderate additional neck pain.

③ I cannot drive as long as I want because of neck pain.

④ It is very difficult for me to drive more than short distances due to neck pain.

⑤ I cannot drive at all due to pain.

Activity and Mobility

⓪ I have complete mobility and can hold my neck in any position without pain.

① I have complete mobility, but holding my neck in a turned position causes pain.

② I have complete mobility but turning my head causes additional pain.

③ My mobility is somewhat limited and pain is increased mildly with movement.

④ My mobility is significantly limited and have severe pain with movement.

⑤ I cannot move my neck due to pain.

Headaches

Pain Intensity

⓪ The pain comes and goes and is very mild.

① The pain is constant and is mild in intensity.

② The pain comes and goes and is moderate in intensity.

③ The pain is constant and is moderate in intensity.

④ The pain comes and goes and is severe.

⑤ The pain is constant and is severe.

Changing Degree of Pain

⓪ The pain is rapidly getting better, or I have no pain.

① The pain fluctuates, but is definitely getting better.

② The pain is getting better, but very slowly.

③ The pain is neither improving nor worsening.

④ The pain is gradually worsening.

⑤ The pain is rapidly worsening.

Reading

- ⓪ I can read as much as I want without a headache.
- ① I can read as much as I want, but it causes a mild headache.
- ② I can read as much as I want, but I need frequent breaks due to headaches.
- ③ I cannot read longer than 1 hour due to headaches.
- ④ I cannot read longer than 1/2 hour due to headaches.
- ⑤ I cannot read at all due to headaches.

Concentration

- ⓪ I can concentrate fully without any difficulty.
- ① I can concentrate fully with minor difficulty.
- ② I have a mild degree of difficulty concentrating.
- ③ I have a moderate degree of difficulty concentrating.
- ④ I have a great degree of difficulty concentrating.
- ⑤ I cannot concentrate at all.

Medication

- ⓪ I never use any medications for headaches.
- ① I use over-the-counter medications less than once a month for headaches.
- ② I use over-the-counter medications regularly for headaches.
- ③ I use prescription medications less than once per month for headaches.
- ④ I use prescription medications regularly for my headaches.
- ⑤ I use prescription medications daily for my headaches.

Frequency and Duration

- ⓪ I have not had any headaches that I can recall.
- ① My headaches are infrequent and very short in duration.
- ② I have about one headache per month.
- ③ I have about one headache per week.
- ④ I have a headache just about every day.
- ⑤ I have a constant headache.

Turn to the next page to score your questionnaire.

Scoring Your Questionnaire

For each of the four parts of this questionnaire, you checked a total of six boxes which corresponded to the statement that was most true for you. Inside of each box that you checked is a number the represents the point value of each statement you checked. Add up your total points for each part and enter them below.

	Mild	Moderate	Severe

General Disability = _____

0 • 2 • 4 • 6 • 8 • 10 • 12 • 14 • 16 • 18 • 20 • 22 • 24 • 26 • 28 • 30

Low Back Pain = _____

0 • 2 • 4 • 6 • 8 • 10 • 12 • 14 • 16 • 18 • 20 • 22 • 24 • 26 • 28 • 30

Neck Pain = _____

0 • 2 • 4 • 6 • 8 • 10 • 12 • 14 • 16 • 18 • 20 • 22 • 24 • 26 • 28 • 30

Headaches = _____

0 • 2 • 4 • 6 • 8 • 10 • 12 • 14 • 16 • 18 • 20 • 22 • 24 • 26 • 28 • 30

Index

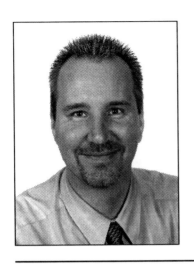

About Dr. Todd Berntson

Dr. Berntson practices in the Minneapolis / St. Paul metropolitan area in Minnesota. He is the author of the book "Why Do I Keep Doing That?" and has had numerous articles published in newspapers, magazines and professional journals. His energy and casual speaking style have made him a popular speaker for a wide variety of seminars and workshops ranging from business groups to social organizations.

Dr. Berntson received his Bachelor of Science in Nutrition from the University of Minnesota and his Doctor of Chiropractic from Northwestern Health Sciences University. He is married to his wife Monique, and enjoys the hobbies of fine art photography and filmmaking.

Dr. Berntson offers entertaining presentations and workshops on exercise, health and the workplace. If you are interested in having him speak at one of your events, please contact him at the following address:

Dr. Todd Berntson
Center Path Media, Inc.
14859 Embry Path
Apple Valley, MN 55124
drtodd@drtodd.com

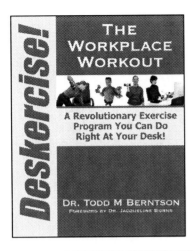

Deskercise!
Order Form

Please mail or fax this form to:

Center Path Media, Inc.
14859 Embry Path
Apple Valley, MN 55124
fax: (651) 407-0803

Name: _____

Address: _____

_____

City: _____ State: _____ Zip: _____

Phone: _____ Fax: _____

Quantity: _____

Subtotal ($21.95 per book): _____

Shipping ($2.50 per book): _____

Total: _____

Payment method:

☐ Check enclosed ☐ VISA ☐ MasterCard ☐ Discover

Name as it appears on card: _____

Card #: _____ Exp: _____ Verification #: _____

I hereby authorize Center Path Media to charge my credit card for the total due for this order.

Signature: _____ Date: _____

Printed in the United States
113241LV00002B/9/A